A Global Portrait of Counselling Psychology

The official birth of counselling psychology is said to have occurred in 1951, when key United States leaders in what was then called the field of guidance and counselling formally adopted the terms 'counselling psychologist' and 'counselling psychology' to describe their profession. In the 65 years that have followed, counselling psychology has thrived, as reflected in the fact that it now is a recognized applied psychology specialty in a number of countries worldwide. The form and expression of counselling psychology differs across countries and yet the specialty retains certain recognizable features wherever it is practiced.

Drawing on data collected through a survey of professionals in eight different countries, this volume considers both ways in which the specialty is distinctive within each of the eight countries, as well as that which is characteristic of counselling psychology across them all. This survey of the international character of counselling psychology examines the emergence and the history of the field; the training, preparation and credentialing of professionals; and the practices and practice settings of counselling psychologists.

This book was originally published as a special issue of *Counselling Psychology Quarterly.*

Rodney K. Goodyear is Professor of Education at the University of Redlands, CA, USA. He is also Emeritus Professor of Education (Counseling Psychology) and former Associate Dean at the University of Southern California, Los Angeles, USA.

James W. Lichtenberg is Emeritus Professor (Counseling Psychology) and former Associate Dean of Education at the University of Kansas, USA.

A Global Portrait of Counselling Psychology

Edited by
**Rodney K. Goodyear and
James W. Lichtenberg**

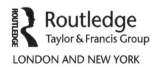

Routledge
Taylor & Francis Group

LONDON AND NEW YORK

First published 2018 by Routledge

2 Park Square, Milton Park, Abingdon, Oxfordshire OX14 4RN
52 Vanderbilt Avenue, New York, NY 10017

Routledge is an imprint of the Taylor & Francis Group, an informa business

First issued in paperback 2019

British Library Cataloguing in Publication Data
A catalogue record for this book is available from the British Library

ISBN 13: 978-1-138-72207-1 (hbk)
ISBN 13: 978-0-367-23401-0 (pbk)

Typeset in Times New Roman
by RefineCatch Limited, Bungay, Suffolk

Publisher's Note
The publisher accepts responsibility for any inconsistencies that may have
arisen during the conversion of this book from journal articles to book chapters,
namely the possible inclusion of journal terminology.

Disclaimer
Every effort has been made to contact copyright holders for their permission to
reprint material in this book. The publishers would be grateful to hear from any
copyright holder who is not here acknowledged and will undertake to rectify
any errors or omissions in future editions of this book.

Contents

CONTENTS

Citation Information

The chapters in this book were originally published *Counselling Psychology Quarterly*, volume 29, issue 2 (June 2016). When citing this material, please use the original page numbering for each article, as follows:

Chapter 1
A global portrait of counselling psychologists' characteristics, perspectives, and professional behaviors
Rod Goodyear, James Lichtenberg, Heidi Hutman, Emily Overland, Robinder Bedi, Kayla Christiani, Michael Di Mattia, Elizabeth du Preez, Bill Farrell, Jacqueline Feather, Jan Grant, Young-joo Han, Young Ju, Dong-gwi Lee, Hyejin Lee, Helen Nicholas, Jessica Jones Nielsen, Ada Sinacore, Sufen Tu and Charles Young
Counselling Psychology Quarterly, volume 29, issue 2 (June 2016), pp. 115–138

Chapter 2
Counselling Psychology in Australia: History, status and challenges
Michael A. Di Mattia and Jan Grant
Counselling Psychology Quarterly, volume 29, issue 2 (June 2016), pp. 139–149

Chapter 3
Counselling Psychology in Canada
Robinder Paul Bedi, Ada Sinacore and Kayla D. Christiani
Counselling Psychology Quarterly, volume 29, issue 2 (June 2016), pp. 150–162

Chapter 4
Counselling psychology in New Zealand
Elizabeth du Preez, Jacqueline Feather and Bill Farrell
Counselling Psychology Quarterly, volume 29, issue 2 (June 2016), pp. 163–170

Chapter 5
Counselling psychology in South Africa
Jason Bantjes, Ashraf Kagee and Charles Young
Counselling Psychology Quarterly, volume 29, issue 2 (June 2016), pp. 171–183

Chapter 6

Counselling psychology in South Korea
Young A. Ju, Young-joo Han, Hyejin Lee and Dong-gwi Lee
Counselling Psychology Quarterly, volume 29, issue 2 (June 2016), pp. 184–194

Chapter 7

Development and current status of counselling psychology in Taiwan
Su-Fen Tu and Shuh-Ren Jin
Counselling Psychology Quarterly, volume 29, issue 2 (June 2016), pp. 195–205

Chapter 8

Counselling psychology in the United Kingdom
Jessica D. Jones Nielsen and Helen Nicholas
Counselling Psychology Quarterly, volume 29, issue 2 (June 2016), pp. 206–215

Chapter 9

Counselling psychology in the United States
James W. Lichtenberg, Rodney K. Goodyear, Heidi Hutman and Emily A. Overland
Counselling Psychology Quarterly, volume 29, issue 2 (June 2016), pp. 216–224

Chapter 10

Counselling psychology's genotypic and phenotypic features across national boundaries
Heidi Hutman, James W. Lichtenberg, Rodney K. Goodyear, Emily A. Overland and Terence J. G. Tracey
Counselling Psychology Quarterly, volume 29, issue 2 (June 2016), pp. 225–233

For any permission-related enquiries please visit:
http://www.tandfonline.com/page/help/permissions

Notes on Contributors

Jason Bantjes is a Counselling Psychologist and Lecturer in the Psychology Department at Stellenbosch University, South Africa.

Robinder Bedi is currently Assistant Professor of Counselling Psychology at the University of British Columbia in Vancouver, Canada.

Kayla D. Christiani, BSc, is a Research Assistant in the Counselling and Psychotherapy research lab at Western Washington University, Australia.

Michael A. Di Mattia is currently a Lecturer in the Faculty of Education at Monash University, Australia. He was National Chair of the Australian Psychological Society's College of Counselling Psychologists (2011–2016).

Elizabeth du Preez is currently a Senior Lecturer, Department of Psychology, Auckland University of Technology, New Zealand.

Bill Farrell is currently a Research Associate, HES Faculty, Auckland University of Technology, New Zealand.

Jacqueline Feather is currently a Senior Lecturer in Psychology, Auckland University of Technology, New Zealand.

Rodney K. Goodyear is Professor of Education at the University of Redlands, CA, USA. He is also Emeritus Professor of Education (Counseling Psychology) and former Associate Dean at the University of Southern California, Los Angeles, USA.

Jan Grant is currently an Adjunct Associate Professor, Faculty of Health Sciences, Curtin University, Australia.

Young-joo Han is currently an Associate Professor, Department of General Counseling, Korea Counseling Graduate University, Seoul, South Korea.

Heidi Hutman is currently an Assistant Professor in the Counseling Psychology master's program in the College of Education at Temple University, USA.

Shuh-Ren Jin is a Full Professor in Counseling Psychology in the Faculty of Education, University of Macau, Taipa, China.

Young A. Ju is currently an Associate Professor, Department of Marital and Family Counseling, Korea Counseling Graduate University, Seoul, South Korea.

Ashraf Kagee is a Counselling Psychologist and Professor in the Psychology Department at Stellenbosch University, South Africa.

Dong-gwi Lee is currently a Professor in the Department of Psychology, Yonsei University, South Korea.

Hyejin Lee is currently a Human Resources Consultant, NdyneINC Corp., Seoul, South Korea.

James W. Lichtenberg is Emeritus Professor (Counseling Psychology) and former Associate Dean of Education at the University of Kansas, USA.

Helen Nicholas is currently a Senior Lecturer in Counselling Psychology at the University of Worcester, UK.

Jessica D. Jones Nielsen is currently a Programme Director and Senior Lecturer in Psychology, City University of London, UK.

Emily A. Overland is currently a PhD candidate at the University of Kansas, USA.

Ada L. Sinacore is currently an Associate Professor, Department of Educational and Counselling Psychology, Associate Member of the Institute for Gender, Sexuality, and Feminist Studies, and the Director of the Social Justice and Diversity research lab, McGill University, Canada.

Terence J. G. Tracey is a Professor in the Counseling and Counseling Psychology Program at Arizona State University, USA.

Su-Fen Tu is currently an Assistant Professor, Graduate School of Education, Chung-Yuan Christian University, Taiwan.

Charles Young is currently an Associate Professor and Counselling Psychologist at Rhodes University, South Africa.

A global portrait of counselling psychologists' characteristics, perspectives, and professional behaviors

Rod Goodyear[a], James Lichtenberg[b], Heidi Hutman[c], Emily Overland[d], Robinder Bedi[e], Kayla Christiani[f], Michael Di Mattia[g], Elizabeth du Preez[h], Bill Farrell[i], Jacqueline Feather[h], Jan Grant[j], Young-joo Han[k], Young Ju[k], Dong-gwi Lee[l], Hyejin Lee[m], Helen Nicholas[n], Jessica Jones Nielsen[o], Ada L. Sinacore[p], Sufen Tu[q] and Charles Young[r]

[a]Graduate Department of Leadership and Counseling, University of Redlands, Redlands, CA, USA; [b]Department of Psychology & Research in Education, University of Kansas, Lawrence, KS, USA; [c]Division of Counseling Psychology, University at Albany, Albany, NY, USA; [d]Department of Psychology & Research in Education, University of Kansas, Lawrence, KS, USA; [e]Department of Educational and Counselling Psychology, and Special Education, University of British Columbia, Vancouver, Canada; [f]Department of Psychology, Western Washington University, Bellingham, USA; [g]Counselling and Psychological Services, University of Melbourne, Melbourne, Australia; [h]Department of Psychology, Auckland University of Technology, Aukland, New Zealand; [i]Private Practice, Private Practice, Titirangi, New Zealand; [j]School of Psychology and Speech Pathology, Curtin University, Perth, Australia; [k]Department of Counseling, Korea Counseling Graduate University, Seoul, Republic of Korea; [l]Department of Psychology, Yonsei University, Seoul, Republic of Korea; [m]NdyneINC Corp, Seoul, Republic of Korea; [n]Institute of Health & Society, University of Worchester, Henwick Grove, UK; [o]Department of Psychology, City University London, London, UK; [p]Department of Educational and Counselling Psychology, McGill University, Montreal, Canada; [q]Graduate School of Education, Chung Yuan Christian University, Taoyuan City, Taiwan; [r]Department of Psychology, Rhodes University, Grahamstown, South Africa

Counseling psychologists in eight countries (Australia, Canada, New Zealand, South Africa, South Korea, Taiwan, the United Kingdom, and the United States) responded to survey questions that focused on their demographics as well as their professional identities, roles, settings, and activities. As well, they were asked about satisfaction with the specialty and the extent to which they endorsed 10 core counseling psychology values. This article reports those results, focusing both on areas in which there were between-country similarities as well as on those for which there were differences. These data provide a snapshot of counseling psychology globally and establish a foundation for the other articles in this special issue of the journal.

Super (1955) reported the official birth of counseling psychology (CP) to have occurred in 1951, when key United States (US) leaders, in what was then called the field of guidance and counseling, voted to adopt the terms "counseling psychologist" and "counseling psychology." During the 65 years that have followed, CP has thrived to the extent that it now is a recognized applied psychology specialty in a number of countries worldwide. The form and expression of CP differs across countries and yet, it is also reasonable to assume that the specialty retains certain recognizable features wherever it is practiced. One indicator of a common identity is the International Association of Applied Psychology's Division of Counselling Psychology (DCoP), which was formed in 2002 (Leong & Savickas, 2007).

This issue of the *Counselling Psychology Quarterly* considers both (a) ways in which the specialty is distinctive within each of the eight participating countries, as well as (b) that which is characteristic of CP across them. The issue builds on an existing literature base that in some cases has described CP as a global specialty (Leong, Savickas, & Leach, 2011), in some cases has described counseling psychology within a particular country to other psychologists in that country (see e.g. Bedi et al., 2011; Fitzgerald & Osipow, 1986; Grant, Mullings, & Denham, 2008; Leach, Akhurst, & Basson, 2003; Scherman & Feather, 2013; Young, 2013), and in other cases, has described CP in a particular country to a broader, international, audience (e.g. Seo, Kim, & Kim, 2007; Wang, Kwan, & Huang, 2011; Young, 2013). The 2004 issue of this journal (see Lalande, 2004; Munley, Duncan, Mcdonnell, & Sauer, 2004; Pelling, 2004; Walsh, Frankland, & Cross, 2004) served that latter purpose. But that issue was published over decade ago and focused only on CP in Western countries (Pelling, 2004). This issue includes recent data from multiple countries and regions to provide a cross-national snapshot of the specialty. A particularly unique and significant aspect of this issue is that it is grounded in survey data from the eight represented countries. Narrative accounts about CP in particular countries are important, but are enriched considerably by the availability of data like that which we report here.

In this article we present data about what CPs do and who they are in Australia, Canada, New Zealand, South Africa, South Korea, Taiwan, the United Kingdom (UK), and the United States (US). Each of the eight short articles that follow is structured using a common framework to discuss CP in those countries. The issue concludes with an integrative article that synthesizes the findings across countries and consolidates this global portrait of CP.

The survey

Surveys in all the participating countries contained a common set of questions. Those questions concerned respondents' personal characteristics (gender, age, level and type of training), work settings, professional roles and activities, and theoretical orientations. Other questions pertained to respondents' satisfaction with the specialty and the extent to which they endorsed 10 values as being characteristic of the specialty. The prototype for this survey was one that Kelly (1961) developed for clinical psychologists, which Garfield and Kurtz (1974) subsequently refined, and which Norcross and his colleagues have since used multiple times (for two examples, see Norcross & Karpiak, 2012; Norcross & Prochaska, 1982). Watkins, Lopez, Campbell, and Himmell (1986) adapted that survey to obtain information about the work, beliefs, and attitudes of CPs in the U.S., and *that* study since has been replicated by Goodyear et al. (2008) and then, Lichtenberg, Goodyear, Overland, and Hutman (2014). In conducting the third survey in that sequence, Lichtenberg et al. realized the potential value of collaborating with colleagues in other countries who could use that survey in their respective national contexts and in so doing, make a global examination of CP possible. This issue of *CPQ* is the result of that collaboration.

Employing common questions across versions of the survey in the US has made it possible to track within-specialty changes across time. For example, together, the Watkins et al. (1986), Goodyear et al. (2008), and Lichtenberg et al. (2014) surveys document three decades of both stability and change in CP in the US. Similarly, a common set of questions permits the between-country comparisons of CP that we report here.

The purpose of this article is to present the results of the surveys that were administered in the eight countries. These results provide foundational material for the remaining articles in this journal issue.

Method

Space limitations have constrained the length of all the articles in this issue. One means of keeping this article brief is to report only the procedures that each country employed to obtain data. Information about the participants, as well as specific information about the survey questions, are provided in the Results section.

Australia

Participants were drawn from the Australian Psychological Society's College of Counselling Psychologists, the largest professional organization of counseling psychologists in Australia. An email invitation was sent to full members of the college ($N = 880$), describing the nature and purpose of the research and requesting participation. The email included a URL link to complete the survey online and the survey was open for 3 months, with a further two reminder emails sent, the first a month after the survey opened, and the second two weeks before the survey closed. The total response rate was 28% (253 of 880), with 230 providing sufficiently complete data.

Canada

The Canadian sample was obtained through the Canadian Psychological Association's (CPA) Section for CP's list-serve. Two hundred twenty section members were each sent an email briefly describing the survey and requesting their participation on the online survey. Additionally, paper versions were offered at the CPA's annual convention in June 2014. The sample included 78 completed online surveys and three paper versions, for a 35.5% return rate. Reminder emails were sent once a month for four months.

New Zealand

The New Zealand sample was obtained by the New Zealand Psychological Society Membership Committee, as well as the Department of Psychology at Auckland University of Technology (AUT). Members of the Institute of Counseling Psychology, as well as graduates from the AUT postgraduate program in CP, were emailed with a request for participation which included a brief description of the survey, an invitation to participate, and a URL link to the online survey.

South Africa

Because no complete list of counseling psychologists' email addresses exists and because a postal survey is impractical in South Africa, a snowball sampling method was used. An initial email that contained a URL link to the online survey was sent to members of four informal networks of counseling psychologists, and participants were then asked to forward the same message to any other counseling psychologists they could think of. Data were collected from mid-June to the end of October 2014.

South Korea

The South Korean data were obtained by two methods. First, participation in the survey was solicited from members of the Korean Counseling Psychological Association through its membership office. Through this offline request, 65 participants responded to the survey. Second, an email solicitation was made to 400 Korean counselors and counselor trainees. The number of responses collected was 398. The email solicitation included a brief description of the study and a URL link to access to the survey.

Taiwan

The Taiwan sample consisted of 124 certified counseling psychologists who had obtained at least a master's degree and passed the National Certification Exam. They participated in this survey via the following two ways. First, an email request consisting of a brief description of the survey, a solicitation for participation, and a URL link to the online survey, was sent to the members of Taoyuan Counseling Psychologists Association and several universities' counseling offices. Also, the Taiwan Counseling Psychology Association and Taipei Counseling Psychologists Association posted the survey information on their websites with a direct link to the online survey. One follow-up request was sent to the identified individuals two weeks after the initial email solicitation.

United Kingdom

U.K. participants were recruited through the British Psychological Association's DCoP to take part in the international survey. Specifically members of DCoP who were chartered members and who identified as counseling psychologists were recruited through the DCoP monthly division newsletter. The division newsletter, which is distributed to over 3000 members, consisted of an explanation and description of the purpose of the international survey, an invitation to survey, and instructions on how to participate, directing potential participants to a URL link to the online survey.

United States

The US sample was obtained by the American Psychological Association's (APA) Membership Office, which selected APA Members and Fellows who had (a) received their doctorates in counseling psychology and (b) were members of the Society of Counseling Psychology (APA's Division 17). The Membership Office emailed a request for participation directly to each of those approximately 2000 persons; the email request consisted of a brief description of the survey, an invitation to participate, and a URL link to the online survey. One follow-up request was sent to the identified individuals two weeks after the initial email solicitation.

Results

This results section will be organized into three sections. The first section includes demographic information about the participants; the second, their work settings, roles; and the third, information about their perspectives, beliefs, and attitudes.

Demographic information

This section provides information about gender, age, and training levels for respondents in each country. Although information about racial and ethnic characteristics is important, the salient categories differed so substantially between countries that it was not feasible or appropriate to attempt a tabular report of that information.

Gender

Data in Table 1 show that most CPs are women, regardless of country. Among the eight countries, the lowest proportions of women were in the U.S. and Canada (61% and 61.5, respectively) whereas; the highest proportions were in Taiwan and South Korea (83.9 and 89.3%, respectively).

Age

Table 1 also reports ages, which were quite variable across the participating countries. The countries in which respondents had the youngest average age were South Korea and Taiwan ($M = 37.7$ and 39.0 years old, respectively) whereas the highest average age were found in Australia and the U.S. ($M = 55.1$ and 52.7 years old, respectively).

Highest earned degree

Table 2 provides information on CPs' highest earned degrees by country. Fourteen (6.1%) Australian respondents indicated holding a bachelor's degree as their highest degree. All other respondents had earned at least their master's degree or its equivalent (e.g. a postgraduate diploma). The proportions of respondents who held a doctorate ranged from 100% in the US to 10.9% in South Korea.

Within the category of doctorate, though, there were between-country differences between the proportions that were research-oriented (PhD or DSc) vs. those with an

5

Table 1. Counseling psychologists' gender and age by country.

	Australia		Canada		New Zealand		South Africa		South Korea		Taiwan		UK		US	
	N	%	N	%	N	%	N	%	N	%	N	%	N	%	N	%
Gender																
Female	192	71	48	61.5	37	68.5	183	80.9	334	89.3	104	83.9	108	72.5	214	61.0
Male	60	22	30	38.5	15	27.8	40	17.7	40	10.7	20	16.1	38	25.5	135	38.5
Transgendered	1	.4													1	.
Missing	16	4.5			2	3.7	3	1.3					3	2	1	.3
Age	M	SD	M	SD	M	SD	M	SD	M	SD	M	SD	M	SD	M	SD
	55.1	12.0	50.8	12.2	50.1	12.4	43.5	12.1	37.7	8.5	39.0	8.2	47.9	12.1	52.7	14.2

Notes: Transgendered was not provided as a response option in all countries. UK age results reflect a conversion of categorical to continuous data; Note that the language for this question varied by country and that Canada asked separate questions for biological sex (which is what is reported here) and gender.

Table 2. Highest earned degree by country.

	Australia		Canada		New Zealand		South Africa		South Korea		Taiwan		UK		US	
	N	%	N	%	N	%	N	%	N	%	N	%	N	%	N	%
Bachelors																
BA/BS/BSc	14	6.1														
Masters (or equivalent)																
MA/MS etc.	131	57.0	32	41.0	16	29.6	177	78.3	301	80.1	104	83.9	25	16.8		
PG Dip	18	7.8			27	50.0										
Doctorate																
Doctorate (unspecified)							48.0	21.2								
PhD	38	16.6	41	52.6	6	11.1			41	10.9	20	16.1	16	10.7	323	92.0
DSc					1	.02										
EdD			3	3.8												
PsyD	1	.4	1	1.3											21	6.0
Dpsych	19	8.3											51	34.2	6	1.70
PsychD													21	14.1		
Missing or Other	6	2.6	1	1.3	1	.4			34	9			2	1.3	1	.30

Notes: PG Dip = post graduate diploma; generally comparable to a Master's degree.

emphasis on professional practice (e.g. EdD, PsyD, Dpsych, PsychD). In fact, the majority of the UK CPs with doctorates held professional practice degrees (48.3% of all respondents with a DPsych or PsychD vs. 10.7% of all respondents who held the PhD).

Work settings, roles, and activities

Work settings

Variability between countries in terms of work settings required modifications of the categories provided for this question (see Table 3). As a result, only four work settings were common across countries: University Counseling Centers, Self-employed/Private Practice, University or Professional School Faculty, and K-12 settings. All other responses were coded as "other" (except in the case of the UK where we retained the category of National Health Service because that category accounted for nearly a third of their respondents).

CPs varied between countries in the extent to which they were employed in these settings. For example, the proportion of CPs working in university counseling centers ranged from a high of 28.2% (Taiwan) to a low of 2.1% (UK). The proportion of CPs who were self-employed or in private practice ranged from none in Taiwan, to 47.4 and 47.3% in Australia and South Africa, respectively; this response option was not provided for South Korean respondents. Similarly, the proportion of CPs employed as faculty members in universities or professional schools of psychology ranged from none in Taiwan to 55.7% in the US. Employment in K-12 settings was relatively low (6.3% or fewer) across all countries, with Taiwan being the exception (28.2%).

Primary work role

Table 4 shows that across seven of the eight countries, the majority of CPs reported themselves to be clinical practitioners. The exception was the US CPs. In their case, the most frequently reported work role (41.3%) was that of academician. No work role other than clinical practitioner had an especially large proportion of CPs engaged in it across the participating countries.

Proportion of CPs engaged in key activities

Table 5 reports the proportions of CPs in each country who reported engaging in each of the 11 professional activities. That is, anyone who reported that any proportion of their time was devoted to a particular activity was counted as engaging in it. The far right columns provide the means (Ms) and standard deviations (SDs) for the proportions across the eight countries and then are ordered from the activity in which the greatest proportion of CPs are engaged to the one in which the smallest proportion are engaged.

Overall, most CPs are engaged to some extent in both administration/management and in counseling or therapy. Averaged across all countries, fewer than half were engaged in any of the remaining nine activities, though there were some instances in which CPs in a particular country were more involved in a given activity than was

Table 3. Counseling psychologists' primary work settings by country.

	Australia		Canada		New Zealand		South Africa		South Korea		Taiwan		UK		US	
	N	%	N	%	N	%	N	%	N	%	N	%	N	%	N	%
University Counseling Center	8	3.5	2	2.6	2	3.7	25	11.1	73	23.2	35	28.2	2	2.1	39	12.8
Self-employed/private practice	109	47.4	28	35.9	16	29.6	107	47.3			0	0	30	32.3	47	15.4
University or professional school faculty (any dept)	22	9.5	20	25.6	6	11.1	35	15.4	11	3.5	0	0	12	13.0	170	55.7
K-12 settings	7	3.0	5	6.4	1	1.9	2	.8	17	5.4	35	28.2			1	.3
National Health Service (UK only)													29	31.2		
Other	84	36.5	23	29.5	29	53.7	58	25.5	212	67.7	54	43.6	20	21.5	48	15.7
Total	230	100	78	100	54	100	227	100	313	100	124	100	93	100	305	100

Table 4. Survey participants' primary work role.

	Australia (%)	Canada (%)	New Zealand (%)	South Africa (%)	South Korea (%)	Taiwan (%)	UK (%)	US (%)
Clinical practitioner	67.0	60.3	61.1	67.4	63.3	78.4	52.7	32.8
Administrator	3.0	2.6	3.7	.0	2.9	3.3		10.2
Researcher	1.3	2.6	.0	1.3	1.3	.8		7.2
Academician	4.8	23.0	3.7		1.3	7.3		41.3
Consultant	3.0	2.6	.0	5.3	.5	.8	14.0	2.3
Supervisor	3.0	2.6	1.9	.4	.0	3.3		.7
Other or missing	17.8	6.4	29.6	16.3	30.5	9.8		5.6

Notes: Blank cells indicate that the particular category was not provided as a specific option on the survey. For Canada, Academician includes the combination of two categories used in their survey (academic and teacher/instructor); for the UK, it included combining four of their categories (Lecturer, Professor, Senior Lecturer, and Reader).

typical across the other counties. For example, New Zealand and Australian CPs were especially likely to be involved in the provision of clinical supervision (69.8 and 65.1%, respectively); South Korean and US CPs were more likely to be engaged in teaching than was otherwise typical (62.1 and 69.7% respectively). Also, US CPs were the most likely to be engaged in some research (58.4%), and a substantially higher proportion of South Korean CPs reported engaging in personality and intellectual assessment relative to the other countries.

Career counseling has long been considered the foundation on which the CP specialty developed, at least in the US (Super, 1955). It is interesting, therefore, that relatively few CPs engage in career counseling across countries. The countries with the highest proportions of CPs engaged in it were South Korea, South Africa, and Taiwan (29.8, 24.4, and 21.1% of CPs, respectively).

Time spent on key activities

Table 6 reports results to the question "if you engage in this activity, *how much time* do you spend engaging in it?" If respondents indicated spending no time on the activity, then their information was not used in calculating the proportion in that particular cell. Given the way the results were calculated, it is important to note that the sums for the proportions allotted to the 11 activities for CPs in any given country exceed 100%.

The far right columns provide the grand means (and SDs) across countries, ordered from highest proportion of time given to an activity to lowest amount of time. It shows, for example, that those who indicated that they are engaged in providing any counseling or therapy (from Table 5, this was 76.5% of CPs across all our samples) typically spent 39.1% of their work time engaging in it. Psychotherapy was the most dominant activity in terms of time spent engaged in it. On the other extreme, only 7.6% of CPs engage in neuropsychological assessment (Table 5) and of the few who do, they reported spending only 7.8% of their time engaged in it.

Table 5. Proportion of counseling psychologists who report engaging in key activities, by country.

	Australia (%)	Canada (%)	New Zealand (%)	South Africa (%)	South Korea (%)	Taiwan (%)	UK (%)	US (%)	Across Country Ms and SDs	
									M	SD
Administration/management	93.8	76.9	93.0	88.5	77.2	78.9	81.7	83.0	84.1	6.8
Counseling/therapy	92.8	74.4	90.7	82.8	93.9	97.6	79.5	59.0	83.8	12.8
Clinical supervision	65.1	42.3	69.8	46.5	56	41.5	19.3	52.1	49.1	15.8
Teaching/training	34.4	46.2	39.5	41.6	62.1	56.1	52.6	69.7	50.3	12.1
Consultation	45.5	48.7	45.8	31.8	24.8	79.7	44.1	41.6	45.3	16.1
Research	21.5	53.8	44.2	42.1	33.3	24.4	35.5	58.4	39.2	13.1
Prevention activities (e.g. psychoeducation; outreach; program development)	28.7	34.6	51.2	36.8	44.3	56.1	24.7	25.9	37.8	11.7
Assessment: personality & intellectual	26.8	35.9	39.5	22.4	68.8	17.9	25.0	25.6	32.7	16.2
Career counseling	7.7	7.7	11.6	24.4	29.8	30.1	11.2	10.8	16.7	9.7
Assessment: vocational	11.5	11.5	11.6	24.3	35.5	6.5	3.2	7.9	14.0	10.7
Assessment: neuropsychological	7.2	.0	11.6	9.7	14.5	3.3	2.8	5.9	7.9	4.3

Notes: Canadian data for prevention activities include both the categories of prevention and outreach and consultation and program development.

Table 6. For those respondents reporting spending any time at all on key activities: the percent time they devote to those activities.

	Australia		Canada		New Zealand		South Africa		South Korea		Taiwan		UK		US		Across country Ms and SDs of the Ms	
	M	SD	M	SD	M	SD	M	SD	M	SD	M	SD	M	SD	M	SD	M	SD
Counseling/therapy	52.4	23.7	42.3	25.0	47.3	24.5	48.6	24.9	40.6	22.8	39.8	22.5	39.3	26.2	36.9	27.8	43.4	5.4
Teaching/training	16.3	16.3	27.3	19.2	18.6	22.8	16.2	18.5	14.6	16.8	18.7	18.0	21.0	16.4	31.8	21.2	20.6	6.0
Administration/management	22.5	14.6	18.6	17.0	19.1	14.1	16.0	10.9	24.4	20.5	21.4	17.0	19.9	15.4	23.9	20.3	20.7	2.9
Research	14.0	17.9	21.3	15.8	11.7	8.3	13.3	16.2	14.9	9.8	14.8	14.0	17.9	14.3	26.9	20.3	16.9	5.0
Prevention activities (e.g. psychoeducation; outreach; program development)	9.4	7.3	11.0	7.0	10.8	7.0	8.8	10.2	12.1	9.8	13.7	8.4	18.3	17.0	9.1	11.2	11.6	3.1
Assessment: personality & intellectual	9.4	8.2	18.6	17.0	13.5	12.8	8.4	10.1	11.5	10.2	5.8	4.0	15.0	9.9	15.6	17.1	12.2	4.2
Consultation	14.8	16.5	12.7	11.8	10.4	11.2	8.9	12.3	7.8	4.6	15.4	10.3	16.8	15.7	12.5	14.6	12.4	3.2
Clinical supervision	11.9	8.8	12.7	14.5	9.7	11.1	7.4	7.3	10.5	6.8	14.3	12.4	16.6	16.8	13.6	10.5	12.1	2.9
Assessment: vocational	9.1	10.5	7.9	7.3	8.4	6.3	5.0	8.5	7.6	4.8	10.0	5.3	20.0	10.0	6.4	8.5	9.3	4.6
Career counseling	6.4	4.0	14.5	18.5	11.4	10.5	7.6	11.8	8.6	6.3	4.3	5.4	10.0	.0	7.1	6.2	8.7	3.2
Assessment: neuropsychological	5.6	4.7	.0	.0	8.8	10.6	5.3	13.1	8.4	6.4	4.3	1.5	13.3	6.5	9.1	9.2	7.8	3.1

Notes: Canadian data for prevention activities include both the categories of prevention and outreach and consultation and program development.

Perspectives, beliefs, and attitudes

Theoretical orientation

Psychotherapy theories, no matter how rudimentary (as per the professor-therapists in Strupp & Hadley, 1979), or implicit (Najavits, 1997), provide essential lenses through which therapists view their clients and understand how to intervene to promote change. The importance of theory was affirmed in these surveys in that respondents reported that their theoretical orientations played an important role in guiding their own practice: across all countries, the mean on a 6-point scale, where 6 was high, was 4.45 (*Mdn* for the 8 countries: 4.11).

As Table 7 indicates, the dominant model among CPs was integrative or eclectic (endorsed across countries by an average of 38.2% of the respondents), followed by cognitive or cognitive-behavioral (CBT; 16.5%), and psychodynamic models (8.0%). However, it is notable that within particular models, considerable between-country differences were found. This variability was especially true of CBT, which was endorsed by as few as 2.6% of the CPs (Taiwan) to as much as 27.8% of them (New Zealand). Additionally, Rogerian or person-centered therapy ranged from a low of 0% (New Zealand) to a high of 17.6% (South Korea).

It is also important to acknowledge the emergence of newer forms of therapies. Only the Canadian survey provided post-modern therapies as a response option (7.7% of their total sample). Yet, this category also volunteered a number of respondents who indicated "other" and specified further (especially in Australia, where 2.2% indicated adherence to some version of post-modern therapies).

Professional identity and career choice satisfaction

Collectively, three sets of questions were intended to tap some aspect of respondents' professional identity. The first set concerned the professional designation they used for themselves and the second concerned their levels of satisfaction with both the specialty and the preparation they had for it. The final set concerned the extent to which respondents reported that their work was informed by 10 values that are often ascribed to CP, using a process that is described below.

Professional self-designation

Respondents in six of the countries were asked to indicate the professional designation they would prefer to use in describing themselves. As Table 8 indicates, in four of those six countries, "counselling psychologist" was the most frequently endorsed of the four options. In Canada, though, a higher proportion indicated that they preferred the term "psychologist" (47.45 vs. 20.5% for "counselling psychologist"), and in South Korea, a higher proportion indicated that they preferred the term "Counselor" (59.6 vs. 25.5% for "counselling psychologist"). One caveat in interpreting these findings is that whereas this question was intended to tap the extent to which the individual identified with CP, there are some countries for which regulatory agencies do not permit individual choice in self-designation (hence the South African survey did not include this question).

Table 7. Counseling psychologists' preferred theoretical orientations by country.

	Australia		Canada		New Zealand		South Africa		South Korea		Taiwan		UK		US		Mean % across countries
	N	%	N	%	N	%	N	%	N	%	N	%	N	%	N	%	
Integrative/eclectic	107	46.5	31	39.7	19	35.2	51	22.5	178	47.3	48	36.7	70	47.0	108	30.8	38.2
Cognitive/cognitive-behavioral	34	12.6	19	24.4	15	27.8	41	18.1	27	7.2	3	2.4	30	20.1	67	19.1	16.5
Psychodynamic (neo-Freudian)	23	10.1	2	2.6	1	1.9	29	12.8	37	9.8	20	16.1	3	2	29	8.3	7.9
Rogerian/person-centered	16	7.0	1	1.3	0	0	27	11.9	66	17.6	9	7	3	2.0	12	3.4	6.3
Humanistic	15	6.6	1	1.3	4	7.4	15	6.6	17	4.5	7	6	3	2.0	18	5.1	4.9
Systems	4	1.7	4	5.1	1	1.9	17	7.5	1	1.1	8	6.5			14	4.0	4.0
Sullivanian/IPT	2	.9	2	2.6	0	0	6	2.6	4	1.1	11	8.9			28	8.0	3.4
Existential	4	1.7	2	2.6	0	0	12	5.3	4	1.1	2	2	6	4.0	7	2.0	2.3
Psychoanalytic	4	1.8	0	0	0	0	7	3.1	7	1.9	4	3.2	2	1.3	1	.3	1.5
Behavioral/learning	0	.0	4	5.1	1	1.9	4	1.7	2	.5	0	0	1	.7	8	2.3	1.5
Gestalt	0	0	1	1.3	0	0	4	1.7	7	1.9	3	2.4			1	.3	1.1
Adlerian	0	0	1	1.3			0	0	2	.5	1	.8			2	.6	.5
Post-modern (solution-focused/narrative)	5	2.2	6	7.7	1	1.9	0	0									3.9
Pluralistic													12	8.1			
Other or missing	55	21	4	5.1	5	9.3	12	5.3	21	5.6	8	6.5	14	9	52	14.9	9.5

Notes: A blank cell indicates that this country did not ask about this particular theory. One exception was with respect to Australia, which did not have a category for post-modern therapies, but 2.2% wrote that in as a category and so they are reported. Therapists endorsing pluralism (in the UK survey only) are those who shift theories according to the client (e.g. person-centered with one client, cognitive with another, etc.).

Table 8. Preferred professional designation for self.

	Australia (%)	Canada (%)	New Zealand (%)	South Korea (%)	UK (%)	US (%)
Counseling psychologist	60.4	20.5	37.0	25.5	74.2	51.1
Counselor	1.3	9.0	5.6	59.6	5.4	.3
Clinical psychologist	3.0		11.1	2.1	3.2	2.6
Psychologist	23.0	47.4	24.1	1.1	33.3	36.4
Other	12.3	23.1	22.2	11.7		9.6

Satisfaction with career choice and training

Participants were asked to indicate their levels of satisfaction with (a) their choice of CP as a career, and (b) their graduate training to be CPs, using a 6-point scale, where 6 = *Very satisfied*. As the data in Table 9 indicate, their levels of satisfaction were quite high, though satisfaction with career choice was somewhat higher than with their preparation for that career (overall means of 5.28 and 4.71, respectively). Moreover, these results were relatively consistent across countries, as indicated by the size of the SDs.

Core values

CP would have no reason to exist as a separate specialty if its practitioners did not adhere to a perspective that differentiates them from other mental health professionals. Super (1955) suggested that this perspective concerns a focus on "hygiology" (in distinction to pathology): no matter how dysfunctional a client might be, CPs are concerned with addressing individuals' strengths. But, as well, a number of other values have been suggested as characteristic of CP (see e.g. Gelso, Williams, & Fretz, 2014; Howard, 1992; Packard, 2009; Strawbridge & Woolfe, 2010). For this survey, we identified the 10 most frequently cited values from those writings and asked respondents to "Please rate the extent to which each of these values guides your work as a counselling psychologist," using a five-point scale where 1 = *Not at all* and 5 = *Very much so*.

Table 10 summarizes respondents' ratings of those values, both by country and then with a grand mean for all countries for each of the values. Notably, the focus on people's strengths (i.e. "hygiology") was both the top rated value, and was also the one for which there was the least variability across countries ($M = 4.59$; $SD = .07$). The grand means were used to create Figure 1, which shows the values clustered into three groups on the basis of their mean values and where the breaks in the data seemed to occur. The first and highest rated cluster concerned focusing on clients' strengths and assets, attention to issues of diversity, focusing on person–environment interactions, and maintaining a developmental focus. The second cluster concerned maintaining a social justice focus, using research to inform practice, using both long- and short-term treatments, focusing on prevention, and addressing career issues. Standing by itself as a third category, and rated the lowest, was the value of conducting research.

Table 9. Satisfaction with counseling psychology as a career choice and with graduate training, by country.

	Australia N = 192		Canada N = 77		New Zealand N = 42		South Africa N = 193		South Korea N = 303		Taiwan N = 124		UK N = 125		US N = 370		Across all Countries	
	M	SD	M	SD	M	SD	M	SD	M	SD	M	SD	M	SD	M	SD	M	SD
	5.34	.92	5.17	1.03	5.46	.67	4.98	1.28	5.02	.95	5.34	.86	5.36	.95	5.51	.81	5.27	.20
	4.72	1.14	4.78	.86	4.95	1.06	4.56	1.24	4.09	1.32	4.84	.79	4.73	1.03	4.98	1.01	4.71	.28

Table 10. Level of endorsement of core counseling psychology values by country.

	Australia N = 224		Canada N = 77		New Zealand N = 41		South Africa N = 189		South Korea N =		Taiwan N = 124		UK N = 93		US N = 370		Across Country Ms and SDs	
	M	SD	M	SD	M	SD	M	SD	M	SD	M	SD	M	SD	M	SD	M	SD
Attention to people's assets, strengths, and resources, regardless of degree of disturbance	4.56	.61	4.69	.57	4.46	.64	4.62	.63	4.59	.69	4.68	.63	4.53	.69	4.60	.62	4.59	.07
A focus on diversity, as well as a consideration of sociocultural context and systemic barriers in making sense of an understanding people's experiences	4.26	.85	4.23	.87	4.34	.88	4.44	.70	4.29	.77	4.57	.55	4.18	.86	4.56	.70	4.36	.15
A focus on person-environment interactions rather than exclusively on either the person or the environment	4.08	1.00	4.26	.83	4.44	.78	4.28	.86	4.28	.75	4.69	.78	4.18	.88	4.47	.70	4.33	.19
A focus on developmental issues and developmentally appropriate interventions across the lifespan	4.34	.79	4.18	.81	4.07	.98	4.38	.79	4.27	.8	4.62	.84	4.13	.86	4.38	.80	4.30	.17
A focus on social justice and the necessity, when appropriate, to advocate for just causes that promote the welfare of others	4.01	.90	3.58	1.08	4.15	.76	4.01	.95	3.16	.98	3.47	.81	3.94	.93	4.25	.87	3.91	.25
Drawing on research to inform practice	4.21	.69	4.26	.82	4.20	.78	3.66	.96	3.93	.8	3.65	.8	4.09	.82	3.99	1.02	3.90	.39

(Continued)

Table 10. (Continued).

	Australia		Canada		New Zealand		South Africa		South Korea		Taiwan		UK		US		Across Country Ms and SDs	
	N = 224		N = 77		N = 41		N = 189		N =		N = 124		N = 93		N = 370			
	M	SD	M	SD	M	SD	M	SD	M	SD	M	SD	M	SD	M	SD	M	SD
An emphasis on both long-term and relatively brief interventions[a]	4.00	.89	3.35	.94	3.88	1.05	3.75	1.01	3.66	.89	4.06	.93	3.47	1.02	3.79	1.14	3.74	.25
A focus on preventive interventions	3.65	1.18	3.48	1.05	3.83	1.22	3.81	1.19	3.59	.89	3.77	.51	3.69	1.07	4.03	1.13	3.73	.17
A focus on career-related issues and concerns pertaining to the workplace (e.g., career decision-making, transitions, adjustment, goal setting, exploration, etc.)	3.30	1.13	3.32	1.08	3.10	1.16	3.51	1.17	3.8	.81	4.16	.57	2.93	1.05	3.63	1.16	3.47	.39
Producing research that adds to knowledge of counseling psychology related topics	2.25	1.35	3.18	1.44	2.35	1.48	2.66	1.40	3.26	1.08	3.55	.84	2.77	1.30	3.31	1.45	2.92	.48

Note: 6-point scale.
[a]This question on the Canadian survey asked only about "relatively brief interventions".

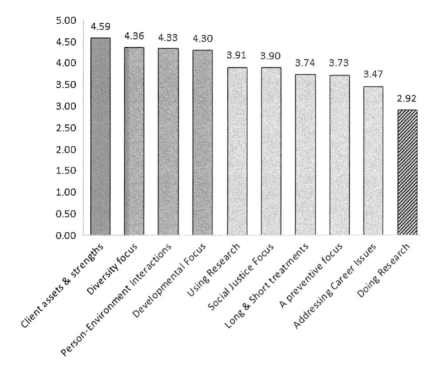

Figure 1. Mean ratings of counseling psychology core values across countries.

Discussion

This issue is important in that it is the first to report data on CPs from around the world. The patterns of the findings and their possible implications will be discussed in the final article in this issue in order to take into account the additional contextual information that is provided in the eight articles that follow. Therefore, we limit this discussion to considerations about sampling and measurement issues that may affect the interpretation of the findings, and which could be helpful in anticipating later global surveys of CP, which we hope will ensue.

This study employed a survey that was derived from one that has been used in multiple iterations in the US over the past 55 years. On the one hand, there are advantages to this sort of continuity across time, especially with respect to the comparisons it permits with prior work. But, there are also possible costs in terms of the extent to which the items are tailored to the unique national contexts in which CPs are working around the world. As well, the field is evolving and the questions should be adapted to address that evolution. One example is evident in the set of questions about theoretical orientation, where narrative and postmodern therapies emerged as having a notable influence on practitioners in the country (New Zealand) that specifically inquired about this form of therapy, and it also emerged as write-in options in other countries. Therefore, we would suggest that in future iterations, collaborations begin sufficiently far in advance that the participating countries could work together to jointly design the questions.

An important issue in interpreting the data presented here is that they were obtained in samples of CPs who were members of professional organizations in their respective countries. But at the same time, there are people who were trained as CPs, but who do not necessarily identify with their specialty through this membership. For example, in the US, the majority of professionals who graduate from CP training programs do not end up becoming members of, or maintaining membership in, the Society for Counseling Psychology. It is reasonable to assume that these individuals would have different employment patterns and attitudes than the members sampled, and there is some evidence to substantiate this conjecture (e.g. Lichtenberg et al., 2014).

It is also important to note that although a broader range of countries is represented in this journal issue than has been true in the past, there are still countries and regions where CPs work that were not included (e.g. Ireland; Hong Kong). For that reason, and because CP is still at the early stages of development in some countries (e.g. China), it is reasonable to expect that a future issue devoted to CP around the world will have a number of additional countries represented.

Finally, these data provide a descriptive snapshot and do not, in themselves, permit statements about factors contributing to differences observed in the data. Some of that information is provided in the richer descriptions of within-country CP, which are provided in the articles that follow in this issue.

Disclosure statement

No potential conflict of interest was reported by the author(s).

References

Bedi, R. P., Haverkamp, B. E., Beatch, R., Cave, D. G., Domene, J. F., Harris, G. E., & Mikhail, A. (2011). Counselling psychology in a Canadian context: Definition and description. *Canadian Psychology/Psychologie Canadienne, 52*, 128–138. doi:10.1037/a0023186

Fitzgerald, L. F., & Osipow, S. H. (1986). An occupational analysis of counseling psychology: How special is the specialty? *American Psychologist, 41*, 535–544.

Garfield, S. L., & Kurtz, R. (1974). A survey of clinical psychologists: Characteristics, activities and orientations. *Clinical Psychologist, 28*, 7–10.

Gelso, C. J., Williams, E. N., & Fretz, B. R. (2014). *Counseling psychology* (3rd ed.). Washington, DC: American Psychological Association.

Goodyear, R. K., Murdock, N., Lichtenberg, J. W., McPherson, R., Koetting, K., & Petren, S. (2008). Stability and change in counseling psychologists' identities, roles, functions, and career satisfaction across 15 years. *The Counseling Psychologist, 36*, 220–249.

Grant, J., Mullings, B., & Denham, G. (2008). Counselling psychology in Australia: Past, present and future – Part one. *Australian Journal of Counselling Psychology, 9*, 3–14.

Howard, G. S. (1992). Behold our creation: What counseling psychology has become and might yet become. *Journal of Counseling Psychology, 39*, 419–442.

Kelly, E. L. (1961). Clinical psychology – 1960. Report of survey findings. *Newsletter: Division of Clinical Psychology of the American Psychological Association, 14*(1), 1–11.

Lalande, V. M. (2004). Counselling psychology: A Canadian perspective. *Counselling Psychology Quarterly, 17*, 273–286. doi:10.1080/09515070412331317576

Leach, M. M., Akhurst, J., & Basson, C. (2003). Counseling psychology in South Africa: Current political and professional challenges and future promise. *The Counseling Psychologist, 31*, 619–640. doi:10.1177/0011000003256787

Leong, F. T., & Savickas, M. L. (2007). Introduction to special issue on international perspectives on counseling psychology. *Applied Psychology, 56*(1), 1–6.

Leong, F. T. L., Savickas, M. L., & Leach, M. M. (2011). Counseling psychology. In P. R. Martin, F. M. Cheung, M. C. Knowles, M. Kyrios, L. Littlefield, J. B. Overmier, & J. M. Prieto (Eds.). *IAAP handbook of applied psychology* (pp. 137 –161). Oxford: Wiley-Blackwell.

Lichtenberg, J. W., Goodyear, R. K., Overland, E. A., Hutman, H. B. (2014, March). *A snapshot of counseling psychology: Stability and change in the roles, identities and functions (2001–2014)*. Presentation at the Counseling Psychology National Conference, Atlanta, GA

Munley, P. H., Duncan, L. E., Mcdonnell, K. A., & Sauer, E. M. (2004). Counseling psychology in the United States of America. *Counselling Psychology Quarterly, 17*, 247–271. doi:10.1080/09515070412331317602

Najavits, L. M. (1997). Psychotherapists' implicit theories of therapy. *Journal of Psychotherapy Integration., 7*, 1–16.

Norcross, J. C., & Karpiak, C. P. (2012). Clinical psychologists in the 2010s: 50 years of the APA Division of Clinical Psychology. *Clinical psychology: Science and practice, 19*(1), 1–12.

Norcross, J. C., & Prochaska, J. O. (1982). A national survey of clinical psychologists: Affiliations and orientations. *The Clinical Psychologist, 35*(3), 1–6.

Packard, T. (2009). The 2008 Leona Tyler Award address: Core values that distinguish Counseling Psychology. *The Counseling Psychologist, 37*, 610–624.

Pelling, N. (2004). Counselling psychology: diversity and commonalities across the Western World. *Counselling Psychology Quarterly, 17*, 239–245. doi:10.1080/09515070412331317611

Scherman, R. M., & Feather, J. S. (2013). Counselling psychology in Aotearoa/New Zealand: Introduction to the special section. *New Zealand Journal of Psychology, 42*, 7–10.

Seo, Y. S., Kim, D. M., & Kim, D. I. (2007). Current status and prospects of Korean counseling psychology: Research, clinical training, and job placement. *Applied Psychology, 56*, 107–118.

Strawbridge, S., & Woolfe, R. (2010). Counselling psychology: Origins, developments and challenges. In R. Woolfe, W. Dryden, & S. Strawbridge (Eds.), *Handbook of counselling psychology* (3rd ed., pp. 3–22). London: Sage.

Strupp, H. H., & Hadley, S. W. (1979). Specific vs nonspecific factors in psychotherapy: A controlled study of outcome. *Archives of General Psychiatry, 36,* 1125–1136.

Super, D. E. (1955). Transition: from vocational guidance to counseling psychology. *Journal of Counseling Psychology, 2*(1), 3–9.

Walsh, Y., Frankland, A., & Cross, M. (2004). Qualifying and working as a counselling psychologist in the United Kingdom. *Counselling Psychology Quarterly, 17,* 317–328. doi:10.1080/09515070412331317585

Wang, L. F., Kwan, K. L. K., & Huang, S. F. (2011). Counseling psychology licensure in Taiwan: Development, challenges, and opportunities. *International Journal for the Advancement of Counselling, 33,* 37–50. doi:10.1007/s10447-010-9111-3

Watkins, C. E., Lopez, F. G., Campbell, V. L., & Himmell, C. D. (1986). Contemporary counseling psychology: Results of a national survey. *Journal of Counseling Psychology, 33,* 301–309.

Young, C. (2013). South African counselling psychology at the crossroads: Lessons to be learned from around the world. *South African Journal of Psychology, 43,* 422–433. doi:10.1177/0081246313504697

Counselling Psychology in Australia: History, status and challenges

Michael A. Di Mattia[a] and Jan Grant[b]

[a]Counselling and Psychological Services, The University of Melbourne, Melbourne, Australia;
[b]School of Psychology and Speech Pathology, Curtin University, Perth, Australia

Counselling psychology in Australia has developed and matured since its emergence in the 1970s. This article provides a brief historical overview and situates counselling psychology (CP) in relation to other applied areas of psychology in Australia. A review of registration, professional organisations, work and role settings and core features is provided. Australian counselling psychologists work predominantly in private practice, as well as hospitals, counselling agencies, universities, medical practices, prisons and government departments. They provide assessment, diagnosis and treatment for mental health disorders and psychological problems related to adverse life events. In addition, they provide couple, family and group therapies. Challenges facing CP in Australia are explored, including a reduction in training programmes, inequities in funding for psychological services and tensions with the definition and description of the scopes of practice.

Development of counselling psychology in Australia

The first discussions about counselling psychology (CP) occurred at the Australian Psychological Society (APS) in 1970 with the Rose Committee report (1970) defining the training and role of counselling psychologists in Australia. It emphasised the importance of reaching all sectors of the population, including those living in the community experiencing adverse life events, as well as those in a clinical setting. Early definitions of CP focused on the need to establish additional services to those provided by clinical psychology (Grant, Mullings, & Denham, 2008). The first training programme in CP commenced in 1975, at La Trobe University. Wills (personal communication, 2015), the inaugural coordinator of the programme, noted that the programme initially focused on school counselling, but soon developed as a programme in psychotherapy, with the curriculum focused on theories of counselling from a variety of perspectives, experiential groups and group therapy, assessment, psychopathology and research methods.

In 1976, the APS Division of Counselling Psychologists was formally established. Its inaugural chair, Williams (1978), noted that one of the early challenges was for CP to establish its own identity and, in particular, to "sort out" its relationship to those other applied areas of psychology where clear overlap existed. He also noted that many members of the newly formed division were influenced by a psycho-educational model of growth, as opposed to a medical model. With the establishment of CP, questions regarding the uniqueness and place of CP in the Australian context (Penney, 1981; Wills, 1980) were further explored during these early years.

In 1983, the Division of Counselling Psychologists became the Board of Counselling Psychologists and in 1993, the current title of College of Counselling Psychologists was adopted. Between 1975 and 2000, six additional CP training programmes developed across a number of other states, with a total of seven programmes in this expansionary period.

Professional associations

The APS is the largest professional organisation representing psychologists, with a membership in excess of 21,000 (for information about APS, see www.psychology.org. au). The APS has nine colleges that each represents one of the recognised areas of practice, including CP. The College of Counselling Psychologists is the largest body representing the professional interests of CP in Australia, with a membership of 1035 (September 2015). The college advocates for CP, internally within the APS, externally to accrediting and regulatory bodies, and politically with government. The college also provides professional development for members, both at a state level and through national conferences. A smaller organisation, the Association of Counselling Psychologists, based in Western Australia, also provides advocacy and professional development opportunities for CPs.

Registration as a CP in Australia

The Psychology Board of Australia (PsyBA) requires all psychologists to be registered after completion of 6 years of training. Three options exist for registration: (1) the completion of 4 years of psychology study at undergraduate level, followed by 2 years of supervised practice and an exam (known as the "4 + 2" pathway); (2) completion of 5 years of psychology study – 4 years at undergraduate level, 1 year of postgraduate study in general psychological practice, followed by 1 year of supervised practice and an exam (known as the "5 + 1" pathway); and (3) completion of 4 years of undergraduate psychology followed by a Masters (2 years), Doctoral (3 years) or PhD (4 years) programme in one of the nine recognised applied areas of psychology.

Becoming a CP requires completion of the third pathway to registration: a Masters, Doctoral, or PhD degree in CP, followed by a period of supervised practice, requiring a minimum of 8 years from commencement of undergraduate studies to completion of the supervised practice. It is then possible for those who have that level and type of training to apply for an *Area of Endorsement* in CP with the PsyBA, allowing use of the title "counselling psychologist."

Accreditation of psychology programmes is undertaken by the Australian Psychology Accreditation Council (APAC), which is appointed by the PsyBA. There are currently two CP postgraduate training programmes accredited by APAC that are taking new enrolments: Curtin University (Perth); and University of Queensland (Brisbane). Three courses, at La Trobe University (Melbourne), Monash University (Melbourne) and Swinburne University of Technology (Melbourne) are in teach-out mode and are no longer enrolling new applicants. In previous years, CP programmes at Macquarie University (Sydney) and the University of Canberra (Canberra) have closed.

CP in comparison to other applied areas of psychology

In Australia, clinical psychology is the dominant area of applied psychology, reflected both in the number of APAC accredited programmes and the total number of psychologists who hold an area of practice endorsement in clinical psychology: 7027, which represents 66% of all psychologists who hold an area of practice endorsement (Psychology Board of Australia [PsyBA], June 2015). In comparison, there are 944 psychologists that hold an area of practice endorsement in CP, the second-largest area representing approximately 9% of all psychologists who hold endorsement.

In 1996, the APS Colleges of Clinical and Counselling Psychologists had almost identical membership: clinical 836, counselling 834 (Martin, 2011). But by 2010, the Clinical College had grown to 3187 members (53% of overall APS college membership), whilst membership of the Counselling College had decreased to 675 members.

Significant changes in the health system occurred during this period which substantially impacted the psychology profession. In 2006, the federal government introduced rebates for psychological services under the *Better Access to Mental Health Care* initiative. This scheme enables people with a diagnosed mental disorder to access 10 sessions of treatment per year from a range of mental health professionals, including psychologists. The demand and uptake for psychological services in the community then increased dramatically and included many people who had not previously accessed mental health care (Pirkis, Harris, Hall, & Ftanou, 2011). However, it has also significantly affected the psychology profession (Littlefield & Giese, 2008). Two categories of services can be provided by psychologists: one for clinical psychologists (*Psychological Therapy* items) and one for all other psychologists (Focused Psychological Strategies [FPS]), who under this scheme are classified as "general" psychologists. This item includes psychologists that have achieved registration through either the "4 + 2" and "5 + 1" pathway, as well as psychologists that possess Masters or Doctoral level qualifications in one of the other eight endorsement areas of applied psychology. The FPS was a term that created for this scheme, for the treatment of mild to moderate high prevalent mental health disorders.

Psychological Therapy items and can only be provided by registered psychologists that hold endorsement as a clinical psychologist with the PsyBA. These items are intended for treating clients with complex and chronic mental health disorders and attract a higher rebate ($125) per 55-min session than general psychology services ($82). However, these items are not restricted to those clients with serious and chronic disorders. Therefore, in practice, clinical psychologists often treat the same high prevalence disorders as other psychologists

This *Two Tiered Model of Funding* has created significant tension in Australian psychology and has afforded clinical psychology greater legitimacy, recognition, and status in Australia and has correlated with the substantial growth of both clinical psychology courses and clinical psychologists. As this has occurred, the number of programmes and psychologists in every other applied area of practice have decreased (Australian Psychological Society [APS], 2012a), resulting in a loss of diversity in the profession.

To illustrate, the numbers of APAC accredited postgraduate psychology training programmes for each of the specialties are (Australian Psychology Accreditation Council [APAC], 2015):

Clinical Psychology	39
Clinical Neuropsychology	6
Community Psychology	1
Counselling Psychology	2
Educational & Developmental Psychology	4
Forensic Psychology	3
Health Psychology	2
Organisational Psychology	8
Sport & Exercise Psychology	1

The financial incentives have skewed student preferences, particularly if a career in private practice is anticipated. Nonetheless, demand for places in CP programmes remains strong (5:1 ratio applicants to places) in those programmes that remain.

Traditionally, clinical psychologists have been employed in public health settings, such as hospitals (Smith & Lancaster, 2000), but have moved in recent years into private practice (Byrne & Davenport, 2005). Many hospitals specifically have written in their Enterprise Bargaining Agreement, that senior positions can be held only by a clinical psychologist or clinical neuropsychologist. This has created difficulties for CPs who work in hospital settings, as career progression is limited. Lancaster and Smith (2002) noted tensions between clinical psychology and CP or clinical neuropsychology in areas of overlap. Clinical psychologists are seen to work with more severe client presentations than CPs, despite the fact that CP programmes focus on psychopathology and psychotherapy for mental health disorders (Brown & Corne, 2004; Grant et al., 2008).

The Better Access scheme has seen private practice become the dominant work setting for psychologists. A survey of Australian psychologists, found 31% of psychologists are employed in independent private practice as their primary occupation, with another 53% employed in private practice as a second job (Mathews, Stokes, Crea, & Grenyer, 2010). The primary roles psychologists report are counselling and mental health interventions, a finding confirmed by Health Workforce Australia (2014), who classifies 81% of psychologists as "clinicians".

Work settings and roles of CPs

CPs are employed in a range of community settings, such as community health centres, hospitals, relationship counselling centres, corrective services, child protection, non-government counselling centres, federal and state police services, veterans' counselling services, university counselling services, and private practice (Grant et al., 2008; Orrum, 2005).

Table 3 in Goodyear et al. (in press) shows that nearly half of Australian CPs are engaged in private practice, as their primary occupation (47.4%). Not indicated in that table is that another 38% are engaged in private practice as a secondary occupation. Eighty per cent of CPs are registered as a Medicare Better Access provider of psychological services and, indeed, the primary role respondents identified (see Table 4; Goodyear et al., in press) was that of clinical practitioner (67%).

This presents a picture of Australian CPs as predominantly private practitioners, engaged in clinical work. However, this shift into private practice has occurred during the last two decades. A 1989 survey found the majority of Australian counselling psychologists were employed in a tertiary setting, either in a university counselling service or as academics, with only 11% employed in private practice (Schoen, 1989).

Core features and traditions of CP in Australia

The training and practice of CP is characterised by a focus on psychotherapy and counselling, diagnosis and treatment of psychological problems and mental health disorders, multiple client modalities, and the therapeutic alliance (Australian Psychological Society [APS], 2012b; Grant et al., 2008).

Counselling and psychotherapy

Knowledge and expertise of counselling and psychotherapy is a core underpinning feature of CP in Australia. Programmes adhere to the scientist–practitioner model (O'gorman, 2001), providing training in a range of evidence-based therapies. Consistent with empirical evidence, which has demonstrated minimal differences in effectiveness between therapeutic approaches (Wampold, 2005; Wampold & Imel, 2015), training programmes teach a range of models, such as cognitive-behavioural, systemic, humanistic-existential and psychodynamic. The survey reflects this eclecticism with 46.5% describing their primary therapeutic orientation as eclectic. This has shifted during the last 15 years, with a survey conducted in 1998 reporting that cognitive-behavioural therapy was the primary theoretical orientation of Australian counselling psychologists (Poznanski & McLennan, 1998).

Diagnosis and treatment of psychological problems and mental health disorders

The ability to treat a wide range of psychological problems and mental health disorders is a key competency requirement for CPs (APS, 2012b). This includes a focus on problems arising from adverse life events, such as loss and grief, relationship difficulties, transition and adjustment issues, through to diagnosed mental health disorders, such as mood disorders, anxiety disorders, eating disorders and personality disorders. In addition, there is a substantial focus on psychopathology, including assessment and diagnosis of mental health disorders.

Whilst CPs are extensively trained to provide counselling and psychotherapy to individuals, training programmes also focus on other modalities. Specifically, they include a focus on couples, group or family therapy, with at least one of these areas extensively covered in the training.

The therapeutic alliance

CP programmes give substantial focus to skills and competence in a range of evidence-based psychological therapies, while concurrently being guided by the empirical evidence supporting the importance of the therapeutic alliance to overall outcome in therapy (Horvath, 2001; Horvath & Bedi, 2002; Krupnick et al., 1996; Martin, Garske, &

Davis, 2000). Emphasis is placed on developing skills in establishing, maintaining and repairing the therapeutic alliance. Programmes are underpinned by both a philosophical and practical emphasis on the importance of evidence-based therapy relationships (Norcross & Wampold, 2011), including the problematic nature of ruptures in the alliance (Safran, Muran, & Eubanks-Carter, 2011).

Issues and challenges for CP in Australia

CP is facing a number of serious challenges and issues, including reduction in training programmes, inequities in Medicare funding and externally imposed definitions of the endorsed area of practice.

Reduction in training programmes

The most pressing issue facing CP is the reduction in postgraduate training programmes. With so few programmes, there are concerns about the future of CP. As discussed above, this is part of a broader issue in Australia, with a number of postgraduate psychology programmes closing in all areas except clinical psychology. Voudouris and Mrowinski (2010) point to several factors that have led to programmes closing. The introduction of the two-tiered Medicare model has led to an increased demand for students wanting to study clinical psychology. However, this has occurred at the same time as federal funding for universities has been reduced, with concomitant pressure on university budgets, leading to the closure of programmes across universities. Postgraduate programmes require small staff–student ratios and intensive teaching and supervision; however, they are underfunded federally, consequently losing an average of $8426 per full-time equivalent student in 2010. When departments are faced with loss-making programmes, they generally reduce the number of postgraduate options available. With the financial pressures facing the university sector in Australia at present, it is difficult to see how new CP programmes (or indeed programmes in any other applied areas) can open in the foreseeable future. With only two active programmes, the challenge for CP is how to now maintain a profile and significance in Australia.

Inequities in Medicare funding

The structure and funding of the *Better Access to Mental Health* care initiative has created difficulties for CPs, as under this scheme they are not permitted to provide *Psychological Therapy*, although this is an acknowledged area of expertise (Australian Psychological Society [APS], 2012c) and an area of core focus for postgraduate CP programmes. The scheme implies that clinical psychologists receive advanced training and are the only group with advanced expertise to deal with chronic and complex mental health disorders, a view promoted by many clinical psychologists. However, CP's frequently work with clients that present with significant and chronic mental health problems. They also receive the same length of training as clinical psychologists and all CP programmes cover psychopathology.

Most respondents in the survey commented on the inequities of the scheme. CP's often work alongside clinical psychologists in private practice settings, with similar client issues, yet receive a significantly lower rebate. This has also affected employment settings, which have begun to adopt this distinction between clinical psychologists and "general psychologists". Unfortunately, this seems to have permeated public attitudes. A survey of the Victorian public found that CP's were seen to be less qualified and skilled, and perceived to work with "normal" client issues (McKeddie, 2013). This suggests there is substantial advocacy and public education work to be done by counselling psychologists to increase understanding of the level of training and expertise they possess.

Definition of CP

With the advent of national registration for psychology in 2010, the PsyBA developed definitions and scopes of practice for the nine areas of applied psychology. Significant tensions exist about the PsyBA definition of CP which, in its (2011) *Guidelines on area of practice endorsements* asserts that "counselling psychologists use their knowledge of psychology and therapy to help individuals develop positive strengths and well-being, and to assist the resolution of problems and disorders" (p. 15). Whilst this is an aspect of the work of CPs it is not the main focus of training or practice. Moreover, it articulates a much more restrictive scope of practice than was established by either the APS College of Counselling Psychologists or the previous Psychologists Board of Western Australia (the functions of which have been taken over by the PsyBA) that emphasised the important role and competencies CPs have in the mental health arena. The APS College of Counselling Psychologists has engaged in significant advocacy to have this definition amended, so far, unsuccessfully.

These difficulties have been exacerbated by extremely vocal and effective clinical psychology advocacy claiming singular and unique expertise in working with mental health disorders. Within Australia, the debates have been extremely acrimonious, in a way that does not seem to have occurred to the same extent in either the US where counselling and clinical psychologists are equally eligible for insurance payments, professional accreditation and employment (Ogunfowora & Drapeau, 2008) or the UK.

Positioning Australian CP into the future

One possibility for the profession to consider is whether to amalgamate areas of practice with common interests at a general level. Martin (2011) has suggested a "super" college in the APS, which could include clinical psychology, health psychology, clinical neuropsychology, CP and forensic psychology, all of which have a common focus on health. Within such a college, there could be divisions and interest groups relating to areas of practice. In this way, CP might have the possibility of preserving its uniqueness as an area of practice.

Such a change would require training programmes to restructure to ensure a focus on core "clinical" skills (consistent with the demand for clinical psychology programmes over the last decade), with options then for students to choose additional subjects that are consistent with more specialised areas of practice. Another model which has been suggested would be for clinical psychology to become the standard core training pathway, with other applied areas offered in the second or third year of postgraduate programmes. This would be a way of ensuring core features of CP continue to be taught in postgraduate programmes. CP needs to continue advocating for equity to deliver *Psychological Therapy* items in the Medicare scheme. If equity were to occur, the desirability of new CP programmes almost certainly would increase.

It is difficult for the public to understand the differences between counsellors, generalist psychologists, clinical psychologists and CPs, despite the different training and standards of psychologists and counsellors. As discussed, becoming a psychologist requires a minimum 6 years of training and mandatory registration with the PsyBA, which is regulated by government. Use of the title "psychologist" is restricted to those that are registered with the PsyBA. In contrast, anyone can use the term "counsellor", as this is not a regulated or protected term. Counsellors do not have a government regulatory or registration body; instead, there are a number of voluntary self-regulating organisations. Counsellors are not eligible for Medicare rebates or for the majority of private health insurance rebates. Therefore, they tend to work in community agencies or to charge lower fees in private practice. Although they may compete in entry level positions in community agencies, CP's generally end up in the supervisory or management positions because of their advanced training. Most government departments and health systems do not employ counsellors, unless they also have registration as a psychologist or social worker. Thus, CP's have more varied and senior employment opportunities. The College of Counselling Psychologists has been extremely active over the last decade in advocacy and public education. It has provided submissions to every major review of mental health, mental health funding, Medicare and insurance commissions. As well, it has challenged statutory bodies over definitions, range of practice and attempts to "water down" the CP mental health competencies. Some of the public education campaign has focused on letters to agencies when positions are advertised that would be suitable for a CP.

The 2015 Counselling College Conference was strategically titled *Counselling Psychologists: Experts in Mental Health*, to emphasise this specific expertise to the public and within the profession of psychology. CPs have had many meetings with both state and federal politicians, including the federal Minister for Health. This advocacy has resulted in some very positive changes, particularly at state level, in overturning discriminatory employment or insurance payment policies. However, further advocacy is necessary for CP to thrive in the future.

Summary and conclusions

Counselling Psychology began in the 1970s in Australia and by the late 1990s there were seven programmes. There are currently two programmes accepting new enrolments. The vast majority of CPs work in private practice as either their primary or secondary work setting, with others working in hospitals, health settings, prisons, government and non-government counselling agencies, university counselling services, academic departments and government departments. This paper has reviewed the number of challenges Australian CPs face, with reduction in training programmes, inequities with funding for psychological services and issues with the definition and scope of the profession. Creative strategies are needed to sustain CP in the future, to ensure it continues to contribute a distinctive and valuable perspective as well as providing expert assessment and psychotherapy services to the public.

Disclosure statement

No potential conflict of interest was reported by the authors.

References

Australian Psychological Society. (2012a). *Psychology 2020. The 2011–2012 presidential Initiative on the future of psychological science in Australia*. Australia: Author. Retrieved June 17, 2015, from http://www.psychology.org.au/Assets/Files/2012_APS_PIFOPS_WEB.pdf
Australian Psychological Society. (2012b). *Competencies of Australian counselling psychologists*. Retrieved May 29, 2015, from http://groups.psychology.org.au/Assets/Files/Counselling%20Psychologists%20Competencies%20-%20December%202012.pdf
Australian Psychological Society. (2012c). *Brochure on counselling psychology*.
Australian Psychology Accreditation Council. (2015). *List of accredited programs*. Retrieved May 29, 2015, from https://www.psychologycouncil.org.au/accreditedcourses/
Brown, J., & Corne, L. (2004). Counselling psychology in Australia. *Counselling Psychology Quarterly, 17*, 287–299. doi:10.1080/09515070412331317567
Byrne, D. G., & Davenport, S. C. (2005). Contemporary profiles of clinical and health psychologists in Australia. *Australian Psychologist, 40*, 190–201. doi:10.1080/00050060500243434
Goodyear, R. K., Lichtenberg, J. W., Hutman, H., Overland, E., Bedi, R., Christiani, K., … Young, C. (in press). A global portrait of counselling psychologists' characteristics, perspectives, and professional behaviors. *Counselling Psychology Quarterly*. doi: 10.1080/09515070.2015.1128396
Grant, J., Mullings, B., & Denham, G. (2008). Counselling psychology in Australia: Past, present and future – Part one. *The Australian Journal of Counselling Psychology, 9*, 3–14.
Health Workforce Australia. (2014). *Australia's health workforce series – Psychologists in focus*. http://www.hwa.gov.au/sites/default/files/HWA_Australia-Health-Workforce-Series_Psychologists%20in%20focus_vF_LR.pdf
Horvath, A. O. (2001). The therapeutic alliance: Concepts, research and training. *Australian Psychologist, 36*, 170–176. doi:10.1080/00050060108259650

Horvath, A. O., & Bedi, R. P. (2002). The alliance. In J. C. Norcross (Ed.), *Psychotherapy relationships that work: Therapist contributions and responsiveness to patients* (pp. 37–70). New York, NY: Oxford University.

Krupnick, J. L., Sotsky, S. M., Simmens, S., Moyer, J., Elkin, I., Watkins, J., & Pilkonis, P. A. (1996). The role of the therapeutic alliance in psychotherapy and pharmacotherapy outcome: Findings in the national institute of mental health treatment of depression collaborative research program. *Journal of Consulting and Clinical Psychology, 64*, 532–539. doi:10.1037/0022-006X.64.3.532

Lancaster, S., & Smith, D. (2002). What's in a name? The identity of clinical psychology as a specialty. *Australian Psychologist, 37*, 48–51. doi:10.1080/00050060210001706666

Littlefield, L., & Giese, J. (2008). The genesis, implementation and impact of the Better Access mental health initiative introducing Medicare-funded psychology services. *Clinical Psychologist, 12*, 42–49. doi:10.1080/13284200802192084

Martin, P. M. (2011). Clinical psychology going forward: The need to promote clinical psychology and to respond to the training crisis. *Australian Psychologist, 15*, 93–102. doi:10.1111/j.1742-9552.2011.0031.x

Martin, D. J., Garske, J. P., & Davis, M. K. (2000). Relation of the therapeutic alliance with outcome and other variables: A meta-analytic review. *Journal of Consulting and Clinical Psychology, 68*, 438–450. doi:10.1037//0022-006X.68.3.438

Mathews, R., Stokes, D., Crea, K., & Grenyer, B. (2010). The Australian psychology workforce 1: A national profile of psychologists in practice. *Australian Psychologist, 45*, 154–167. doi:10.1080/00050067.2010.489911

McKeddie, J. (2013). Profiling a profession: A victorian survey assessing lay attitudes toward and knowledge of counselling psychologists. *Australian Psychologist, 48*, 128–138. doi:10.1111/j.1742-9544.2011.0046.x

Norcross, J. C., & Wampold, B. E. (2011). Evidence-based therapy relationships: Research conclusions and clinical practices. *Psychotherapy: Theory, Research, Practice, Training, 48*, 98–102. doi:10.1037/a0022161

O'gorman, J. G. (2001). The scientist-practitioner model and its critics. *Australian Psychologist, 36*, 164–169. doi:10.1080/00050060108259649

Ogunfowora, B., & Drapeau, M. (2008). Comparing counseling and clinical psychology practitioners: Similarities and differences on theoretical orientations revisited. *International Journal for the Advancement of Counselling, 30*, 93–103. doi:10.1007/s10447-008-9048-y

Orrum, M. (2005). *Counselling psychologists in Western Australia: Roles, functions, settings, and professional identity* (Unpublished master of psychology dissertation). Curtin University, Perth.

Penney, J. F. (1981). The development of counselling psychology in australia. *Australian Psychologist, 16*, 20–29. doi:10.1080/00050068108254412

Pirkis, J., Harris, M., Hall, W., & Ftanou, M. (2011). *Evaluation of the Better Access to Psychiatrists, Psychologists and General Practitioners through the Medicare Benefits Schedule initiative: Summative evaluation*. Melbourne: Centre for Health Policy, Programs and Economics.

Poznanski, J., & McLennan, J. (1998). Theoretical orientations of Australian counselling psychologists. *International Journal for the Advancement of Counselling, 20*, 253–261. doi:10.1023/A:1005389228647

Psychology Board of Australia. (2011). *Guidelines on area of practice endorsements*. Retrieved June 7, 2015, from http://www.psychologyboard.gov.au/StandardsandGuidelines/Codes-Guidelines-Policies.aspx

Psychology Board of Australia. (2015). *Psychology registrant data: June 2015*. Retrieved August 20, 2015, from http://www.psychologyboard.gov.au/About/Statistics.aspx

Rose, D. E. (1970). *The professional training of counselling psychologists* (Reports of Standing Committee on Training). Australia: Australian Psychological Society.

Safran, J. D., Muran, J. C., & Eubanks-Carter, C. (2011). Repairing alliance ruptures. *Psychotherapy, 48*, 80–87. doi:10.1037/a0022140

Schoen, L.G. (1989). In search of a professional identity: Counseling psychology in Australia. *The Counseling Psychologist, 17*, 332–343. doi:10.1177/0011000089172011

Smith, D., & Lancaster, S. (2000). The practice of clinical psychology in Victoria, part 1: Where they work and what they do. *Clinical Psychologist, 5*, 27–32. doi:10.1080/13284200108521075

Voudouris, N., & Mrowinski, V. (2010). Alarming drop in availability of postgraduate psychology training. *InPsych, 32*, 20–23.

Wampold, B. E. (2005). Establishing specificity in psychotherapy scientifically: Design and evidence issues. *Clinical Psychology: Science and Practice, 12*, 194–197. doi:10.1093/clipsy.bpi025

Wampold, B. E., & Imel, Z. E. (2015). *The great psychotherapy debate. The evidence for what makes psychotherapy work* (2nd ed.). New York, NY: Routledge.

Williams, C. (1978). The dilemma of counselling psychology. *Australian Psychologist, 13*, 33–40. doi:10.1080/00050067808415564

Wills, G. (1980). An examination of the relationship between counselling and counselling psychology. *Australian Psychologist, 15*, 73–84. doi:10.1080/00050068008254372

Counselling Psychology in Canada

Robinder Paul Bedi[a], Ada L. Sinacore[b] and Kayla D. Christiani[c]

[a]Faculty of Education, ECPS, University of BC, Vancouver, British Columbia, Canada; [b]Department of Educational and Counselling Psychology, and Special Education, University of British Columbia, Department of Psychology, Western Washington University, Bellingham, WA, USA; [c]Department of Educational & Counselling Psychology, McGill Univ, Montreal, Canada

Counselling psychology in Canada has experienced tremendous growth and greater recognition within the last 30 years. However, there is little empirical research on the practice of counselling psychology in Canada and the characteristics of Canadian counselling psychologists. We administered a 74 item questionnaire to 79 counselling psychologists who were members of the Counselling Psychology Section of the Canadian Psychological Association, achieving a 35.4% response rate. The survey asked various questions organized under the headings of: Background Information, Theoretical Orientations, Professional Activities, Training and Career Experiences, and Future. Overall, these Canadian counselling psychologists seem to see the discipline as moderately different from clinical psychology and from counsellor education, and are largely satisfied with their choice of career in counselling psychology. Results further indicate that independent practice is the most common work-setting and that respondents spend a large share of their time providing individual, non-career related, counselling/psychotherapy of primarily a rehabilitative/treatment-oriented nature. A strengths-focused approach was also highly valued by the sample. The development of the field, distinctive characteristics of Canadian counselling psychology, the place of counselling psychology in the Canadian health care delivery system, credentialing, professional organizations, education and training issues, allied professions, opportunities for the field, and threats to the field are also discussed.

Counselling psychology in Canada has experienced tremendous growth and greater recognition within the last 30 years. This article offers an overview of counselling psychology in Canada grounded in a 2014 survey of counselling psychologists. We administered a 74-item questionnaire to 79 counselling psychologists who were full or fellow members of the Section of Counselling Psychology (SCP) of the Canadian Psychological Association (CPA) – the national association of psychology in Canada – and who possessed at least a master's degree. The survey asked various questions organized under the headings of: Background Information, Theoretical Orientations, Professional

Table 1. Demographics for sample.

Characteristic	N	%
Gender		
Masculine	30	38.5
Feminine	47	60.3
Other	1	1.3
Sexual orientation		
Heterosexual	73	93.6
Gay	4	5.1
Queer	1	1.3
Ethnic origin		
European	56	71.8
Asian	6	7.7
Canadian	5	6.4
Aboriginal/Caribbean/African	3	3.9
Multi-ethnic	5	6.4
Other	3	3.9
Citizenship		
Canadian	71	94.7
British/Hong Kong/United States	4	5.2
Birthplace		
Canada	56	72.7
United States	8	10.3
Other	13	16.9

Note: Some demographics may add up to 99.9 or 100.1% (due to rounding).

Activities, Training and Career Experiences, and Future. About 96% of the sample completed an online version of the survey while the remaining completed paper copies available during the 2014 convention of the CPA. Respondents were offered a $15 gift card for participation. We achieved a 35.4% response rate and received responses from 10 out of the 13 provinces and territories of Canada. Demographic information about the sample is provided in Table 1 (see also Goodyear et al., in press, Tables 1–3).

Development and evolution of counselling psychology in Canada

Counselling psychology as a formal discipline in Canada was started by a small group of scholars at Memorial University (Sinacore, 2015). These individuals crafted a petition for the development of the SCP within the CPA (Hurley, 2010; see also Friesen, 1983). In 1986, this request was approved by the CPA executive and, in 1987, the SCP held its first business meeting at the CPA Annual Convention with M. Schoenberg as the first Chair of the SCP (Schoenberg, 1988). Subsequently, the SCP grew from an initial membership of 27 in 1987 (Hurley, 2010) to over 450 members (including student members) currently.

Prior to the development of the SCP within the CPA, many of the early pioneers belonged to and continued to belong to the Canadian Counselling and Guidance Association (now called the Canadian Counselling and Psychotherapy Association [CCPA]), particularly to the Counsellor Educator Chapter, as they were generally involved in training counsellors (Lalande, 2004). Thus the development of counselling psychology in Canada is rooted in both the disciplines of professional counselling and professional psychology (Lalande, 2004) but emerged primarily out of the counselling profession rather than through the applied psychology profession (Hiebert & Uhlemann, 1993; Young & Nicol, 2007).

A major landmark for the field occurred in 2009. After an extensive consultation process, comprehensive literature reviews, and careful analyses of materials from local counselling psychology associations and training programmes, the SCP Definition Committee (co-chaired by Robinder P. Bedi and Beth E. Haverkamp) developed a Canadian definition of counselling psychology which was subsequently adopted by the CPA (Beatch et al., 2009). A year after the definition was adopted, Ada L. Sinacore conceptualized and chaired the *Inaugural Canadian Counselling Psychology Conference* (ICCPC). The aim of the conference was to "document the history of Canadian counselling psychology, identify the current state of the discipline and conceptualize future directions for growth" (see http://www.mcgill.ca/inauguralccpc). The conference resulted in a range of concrete outcomes which included the establishment of an SCP Archive Committee, the publishing of the first Special Section on Counselling Psychology in the journal *Canadian Psychology* (Guest Editor Ada L. Sinacore) and a co-edited book (Sinacore, 2015) entitled, *Canadian Counsellors and Counselling Psychologists in the twenty-first Century,* the first book devoted to Canadian counselling psychology and counselling.

Credentialing

Registration as a psychologist in Canada is a provincial/territorial responsibility with notably different standards across the country. One does not get licensed specifically as a counselling psychologist but rather as a "registered psychologist" although some provinces allow the psychologist to declare counselling psychology as a specific area of practice. Whereas the CPA advocates for a doctoral degree as the national standard for registration as a psychologist, only about half of the provinces/territories require a doctoral degree for registration. In addition, the Canadian and provincial governments are advocating that all psychologists registered in one province/territory should be eligible for a license in anywhere in the country. Although these laws are in place, full and consensual procedures to implement them are still under development and much opposition still exists due to largely disparate requirements across provinces and territories (see http://www.cpa.ca/practitioners/practiceregulation/). Alternately, in several provinces where a doctoral degree is required, one may still register with the provincial college with a master's degree in psychology and appropriate coursework and supervised training as a "psychological associate" rather than a psychologist.

A very recent development is the registration of master's level practitioners outside of psychology provincial regulatory bodies and through regulatory colleges more associated with counsellors and psychotherapists. The province of Ontario offers a license as a psychotherapist through the College of Psychotherapists (and, at the same time, offers a license as a Psychological Associate through the College of Psychologists). In the province of Quebec, a Master's-level counsellor can hold a license as a Conseillères d'Orientation (Guidance Counsellor). Nova Scotia also has a Master's-level license which is regulated by the Nova Scotia College of Counselling Therapists. Otherwise, the profession of counselling remains unregulated in the rest of Canada at the time of writing this article.

This variety of licensure opportunities was partially reflected in our sample of SCP members as 74.4% maintained registration as a psychologist but 6.4% did also or instead as a psychotherapist, 5.1% as a psychological associate, 5.1% as a counselling therapist, 2.6% as a guidance counsellor and 6.8% maintained some other professional license or registration. In addition, in Canada, the Canadian Counselling and Psychotherapy Association (CCPA) offers a national certification as a Canadian Certified Counsellor to its members who meet additional standards although only 16.7% of the respondents to our survey held this credential.

Place of counselling psychology in the Canadian health care delivery system

Although Canada has a publically funded national health care system, for the most part, psychological services are not comprehensively covered outside of hospitals, schools/ academic institutions, and correctional facilities. Based on the results of our survey, it appears that the majority of Canadian counselling psychologists work in either independent practice or as part of an academic university department. Holding multiple positions is common with most involved in independent practice in some way, as either their primary, secondary or tertiary position. The prevalence of independent practice work is not surprising as psychology services are not extensively covered under Canada's national health care system as noted already so, given the great demand and the extremely limited free public services available, most individuals rely on private insurance plans in order to access a psychologist. However, affordability and lack of access are still significant problems as even those who have private supplemental health care insurance often face severe limits on coverage (Domene & Bedi, 2013).

Professional organizations

The CPA is the national association for psychology in Canada with over 7000 members (see 2015 annual report of the CPA available at: http://www.cpa.ca/aboutcpa/annualgen eralmeetingsandreports). As noted on its website (http://www.cpa.ca), its objectives include the promotion of excellence in psychological research, education, and practice as well as the promotion of the advancement, development, dissemination, and application of psychological knowledge. The CPA currently maintains 34 sections (including the SCP) to promote specific interests within the broader field of psychology. The SCP is the third largest section behind the Student Section and the Section of Clinical Psychology (Bedi et al., 2011). It currently maintains close to 450 members including about 200 student members (see http://www.cpa.ca/aboutcpa/annualgeneralmeetingsan dreports). Based on these numbers, it is pretty evident that the vast majority of Canadian counselling psychologists do not belong to the SCP. For those who were members of the SCP and responded to our survey, a notable but small proportion also belonged to the Section of Clinical Psychology (14.1%), Section of Aboriginal Psychology (11.5%), and Section on Traumatic Stress (8.9%). About 15% of our sample also maintained affiliation with the American Psychological Association (APA) and about 19% maintained affiliation with the CCPA. The CCPA is a 5000 + member national organization that promotes the counselling profession by providing leadership, education, advocacy and professional development to counsellors and psychotherapists, and predominantly represents Master's-level counsellors/psychotherapists and counsellor

educators (see http://www.ccpa-accp.ca/ and http://www.ccpa-accp.ca/annual-financial-re
ports/) although there are a number of prominent counselling psychologists very active
in this organization.

Accredited education and training in counselling psychology

Educational programmes

The CPA currently accredits doctoral programmes in clinical, counselling and school
psychology programmes under the same guidelines, while there are unique guidelines
for the accreditation of clinical neuropsychology programmes. Accreditation of counselling psychology doctoral programmes began in 1989 at the request of the SCP
(Lalande, 2004) at which time the SCP was asked to adopt the accreditation criteria and
procedures of the Section on Clinical Psychology (Young & Lalande, 2011). However,
there were concerns that the common accreditation procedures would compromise the
unique professional identity of counselling psychology (Sinacore, 2015; Sinacore et al.,
2011). In 2006, the SCP struck an ad hoc committee that provided formal recommendations for revising the standards such that they would be more inclusive of counselling
psychology core values such as multiculturalism, social justice and qualitative research
(Sinacore, 2015).

Currently, there are five CPA-accredited doctoral programmes in counselling psychology (University of British Columbia, University of Alberta, University of Calgary,
McGill University and the University of Toronto), 26 in clinical psychology, two in
school psychology, and one in clinical neuropsychology. All five programmes in counselling psychology subscribe to the scientist–practitioner model of training and only
offer PhD degrees. Unlike virtually all clinical psychology programmes in Canada (who
admit students with a bachelor's degree who complete their master's and doctoral work
in the same university and psychology department with reserved spaces for admission
to the doctoral programme upon successful completion of the master's), they are not
integrated master's/doctoral programmes and require a master's degree in counselling,
counselling psychology or related field for admission. It is extremely common for counselling psychologists in Canada to complete their master's and doctoral degrees at
different universities (Bedi, Klubben, & Barker, 2012).

The number of CPA-accredited counselling psychology doctoral programmes in
Canada has remained relatively stable with the latest addition (the University of
Calgary) coming in 2010. The first accredited programme (McGill University) achieved
this recognition in 1999, followed by the University of Alberta and the University of
British Columbia in 2000. The University of Toronto received it in 2006. To our knowl-
edge no doctoral programmes are currently in the process of seeking accreditation.

Prior to August 2015, the APA also accredited doctoral programmes in Canada and
two Canadian counselling psychology programmes had maintained APA-accreditation.
While, the effects of the loss of APA accreditation to Canadian programmes is not yet
fully known, it is hoped that the *First Street Accord* between APA and CPA which rec-
ognizes the equivalency of the two systems of accreditation (http://www.apa.org/ed/ac
creditation/first-street-accord.aspx), will allow an ease of cross-border movement for
counselling psychologists and counselling psychology doctoral students.

Graduation from an accredited programme is not a prerequisite to seeking provincial registration as a psychologist or declaring counselling psychology as an area of practice. Of those with doctoral degrees in our sample, 28.9% graduated from CPA-accredited doctoral programmes, 13.3% from APA-accredited programmes, 35.6% from programmes that were accredited by both CPA and APA, and 22.2% from non-accredited programmes. Our respondents also held master's degrees in counselling psychology (55.3%), clinical psychology (15.8%), counselling/counsellor education (6.6%), and educational psychology (6.6%), or some other area (totalling 15.7%). At present, there are only three universities with master's programmes in professional counselling accredited by the CCPA, two of which were accredited relatively recently. Thus it is safe to assume that the vast majority of counselling psychologists first obtained master's degrees from non-accredited master's programmes.

Internship training programmes

CPA accreditation for counselling psychology programmes requires that students complete a minimum 1600-h internship centred on supervised practice (Haverkamp, Robertson, Cairns, & Bedi, 2011). In Canada, there are 3 accredited internships that specifically identify as counselling psychology sites and a small number that will accept both clinical and counselling psychology students. With approximately 25 counselling psychology doctoral students requiring an internship placement each year, there is a severe shortage of accredited internship sites (Haverkamp et al., 2011). The challenge of securing an accredited internship was particularly highlighted in the survey of SCP members. That is, while 74.4% of respondents stated that they completed a doctoral-level internship, only 15.4% completed an APA-accredited internship and 14.1% a CPA-accredited internship. In other words, most completed a non-accredited internship. The most common sites in which doctoral-level internships were completed included: hospital/medical centres (35.3%), university counselling centres (33.0%), and community mental health clinics/agencies (9.8%).

Allied disciplines and professions

The two disciplines with the most overlapping training and scope of practice with counselling psychology in Canada are professional counselling and clinical psychology (Beatch et al., 2009). This is partly reflected in the results of the survey whereas some members of the SCP possessed doctoral degrees in areas other than counselling psychology, including: clinical psychology (17.8%), educational psychology (8.9%) and counselling/counsellor education (6.7%).

Given the existence of both the CPA and CCPA and the emergence of counselling psychology through the efforts of counsellor educators, a common concern is confusion between counsellor education and counselling psychology and how to be allied but distinct disciplines (Bedi et al., 2011). This is compounded by counselling psychologists sometimes playing prominent roles in the CCPA Counsellor Educator Chapter, by the existence of PhDs geared towards counsellor education, and because counsellor educators often teach in counselling psychology PhD programmes in Canada. Given virtually identical accreditation standards and highly overlapping scopes of practice (Linden, Moseley, & Erskine, 2005), much confusion also remains between counselling psychology and clinical psychology (Bedi et al., 2011). These points are clearly reflected in our survey as respondents rated the field of counselling psychology as moderately distinctive from the field of professional counselling on average with 3.9% stating "not at all" and 15.8% stating "very much so." They also rated counselling psychology as only moderately distinctive from clinical psychology overall with 6.5% saying "not at all" and 14.3% saying "very much so." Furthermore, respondents saw the practice of professional counselling (traditionally associated with counsellors and counselling psychologists) as only slightly different from the practice of psychotherapy (traditionally associated with clinical psychologists and psychiatrists) overall with 22.4% reporting "not at all" and 9.2% reporting "very much so."

Traditions and characteristics of canadian counselling psychology

Values

As noted earlier, counselling psychology obtained its first nationally endorsed consensual definition in 2009. The definition (available at http://cpa.ca/aboutcpa/cpasec tions/counsellingpsychology; see Bedi et al., 2011) highlights the discipline's commitment to health, wellness, remediation, prevention, psychoeducation and advocacy. It also highlights its orientation to collaborative, developmental and multicultural models, as well as its focus on transitions across the life span. Additionally, the definition identifies key core values of Canadian counselling psychology: taking a strength based, client centred, and holistic approach to assessment, diagnosis and case conceptualizing while attending to social, cultural, familial and contextual factors. Finally, the definition emphasizes the intersection of research and practice with a clear statement to the importance of conducting both qualitative and quantitative research that are culturally appropriate. As noted by Goodyear et al. (2016a), the most strongly endorsed value in our sample by far was "attention to people's assets, strengths and resources, regardless of degree of disturbance" and this value also maintained the lowest variability of ratings across our sample. Of the values surveyed, the lowest rated ones were related to producing research and a focus on career and workplace issues (see Goodyear et al., 2016a) and the largest variability across respondents were for endorsement of the values related to producing research, career, prevention and social justice.

Work identity and settings

As noted by the definition cited above and supported by the survey results, Canadian counselling psychologists self-identify in many ways and work in a multitude of settings. The majority of participants described themselves to others using the professional label of psychologist (47.5%), counselling psychologist (20.5%), therapist/psychotherapist (11.5%) or counsellor (9.0%). As well, they identified the following professional work identities: 60.3% of respondents listed their primary work role as "practitioner" followed by 20.0% as "academic." For secondary identity, the highest values were: "consultant" (26.3%), "teacher/instructor" (23.7%), "researcher" (16.7%), "practitioner" (10.5%), "supervisor" (9.2%), "administrator" (7.9%) and "academic" (5.7%).

Our results also indicated that holding multiple positions was common, as respondents indicated that they worked an average of 39.6 h per week (SD = 12.8) at their primary job and those who worked a second job (61.0%) added an average of 7.2 h per week (SD = 6.9). About 23.3% held a third job, working an average of 1.6 additional hours per week (SD = 2.9). As noted by Goodyear et al. (2016a, Table 3), in terms of primary work setting, the most common setting (35.9%) was independent practice, followed by a position in a university academic department (25.6%), usually in an education/counselling department rather than a department of psychology. About 10% of respondents worked in a community agency. Very few (less than 5% each) worked in alternative settings such as a university counselling centre, K-12 school setting, corporate/business setting, forensic/correctional setting, psychiatric hospital, outpatient health centre, hospital, government setting and rehabilitation centre. The most common secondary work settings were independent practice (58.3%) or community agency (8.3%). The only third work setting endorsed by more than one respondent was independent practice. When disaggregating primary work setting by biological sex, men were found to work more frequently in a university department whereas women were found to work more frequently in independent practice : χ^2 (4) = 9.3, p = 0.05) with a small effect size of Cramer's V = 0.25.

Professional activities

Canadian counselling psychologists appear to be an incredibly diverse group in terms of services offered with huge variability in how they spend their work week (see Goodyear et al., 2016a, Tables 5 and 6). They spend the most professional time on administration/management and counselling/therapy, and about half are involved, currently and in some way, in research. This latter finding could be due to the fact that all doctoral programmes in counselling psychology are contained within research-intensive universities, over a quarter of our respondents had their primary position in a university academic department, and many listed their secondary or tertiary positions at a university (presumably as primarily teaching or serving on student research committees or both). Regardless, amongst those who provide counselling/psychotherapy services, most of their time is spent providing treatment-oriented services (M = 45.4%, SD = 34.3) rather than developmental (M = 34.1%, SD = 27.9) or preventative (M = 20.5%, SD = 19.5) services with individual counselling/ psychotherapy being, by far, the most frequent modality used (M = 77.7%, SD = 18.6), followed by couples counselling/psychotherapy (M = 10.0%, SD = 12.0), family counselling/psychotherapy (7.5%, SD = 12.8), and group counselling/psychotherapy (M = 4.8%, SD = 10.9). Career counselling was only done by 7.7% of the sample and vocational assessment was only provided by 11.5% of the sample. Even the small amount of counselling psychologists who provided either of these services spent only a very small minority of their time engaged in them.

Theoretical orientation

Respondents indicated that their theoretical orientation "often" affected their practice. Like in most countries examined (see Goodyear et al., 2016a, Table 7), the most common primary theoretical approach was eclectic/integrative followed by cognitive-behavioural. Post-modern theoretical approaches were ranked third in Canada followed by Systems theories and Behaviourism. About 21.8% of respondents indicated that their secondary orientation was eclectic/integrative, followed by Rogerian/person-centred

(15.4%), post-modern (11.5%), existential (6.4%), systems (5.1%), and behavioural/learning (3.8%). For those who defined their primary or secondary theory as eclectic/integrative, 50.0% endorsed theoretical integration, 41.3% endorsed technical eclecticism, and 8.7% indicated atheoretical or had no preferred manner of integration.

Opportunities and threats
Opportunities
The SCP has had steady membership growth since it was founded. As well, there are over 40 master's level counselling or counselling psychology programmes which provide a large and steady pool of applicants for PhD programmes in counselling psychology (Bedi et al., 2012). In addition, over the last few years, there is a slightly increasing number of accredited internship sites accepting counselling psychology students and there are consistent efforts to increase the number specifically devoted to counselling psychology practice. As such, it is safe to say that the discipline remains strong in Canada with ongoing efforts to ensure its prosperity in the future, especially in serving a diverse population.

Canada is a very linguistically, religiously and ethnically diverse country with one of the highest per-capita immigration rates in the world; providing ample opportunities to develop and demonstrate cross-cultural and multicultural competence – two areas of strength endemic to the Canadian definition of counselling psychology and two areas where several Canadian counselling psychologists have conducted nationally acclaimed research (Domene & Bedi, 2013). We expect Canadian counselling psychologists to continue to play a leadership role in researching topics like acculturation and providing services to populations such as immigrants and refugees (Domene & Bedi, 2013; see also Bedi & Domene, 2015).

Threats
As is probably the case with many professions, there seems to be an upcoming high level of professional turn-over. About 35% of our survey respondents are either retiring or leaving the profession within the next 5 years, which may pose a challenge to the growth and continued vitality of the field if these positions are not filled by counselling psychologists. However, the biggest threats to Canadian counselling psychology, in our opinion, pertain to distancing itself from its historical strengths and defining areas (e.g. career counselling, training and working in university counselling centres) and the continuing clouding of professional identity.

Career counselling and career assessment, considered historically foundational to the discipline (Young & Nicol, 2007), are not offered regularly on a weekly basis by over 90% of participants in our sample. That is, although the roots of Canadian counselling psychology are in educational and career counselling (Young & Nicol, 2007), the field now appears to be moving away from these positive psychology, developmental, preventative and person-environment-fit roots (Linley, 2006). This movement is consistent with the findings of this study, wherein Canadian counselling psychologists now work, with notable frequency, in hospitals, correctional facilities, and other non-traditional settings rather than just in settings that long characterized the profession (e.g. counselling centre).

Although it has long been assumed that university counselling centres serve as key cornerstone of supervised training for counselling psychology students (Bedi et al., 2011), results of our survey indicate that as many if not more counselling psychology doctoral students now complete their internships in a hospital-setting – a location premised on a medical model of psychological services with mental health services provided mostly by psychiatrists, clinical psychologists and psychiatric nurses. Thus, there is a likelihood that training in these sites has negative consequences for professional identity development as a counselling psychologist (Haverkamp et al., 2011). Yet, part of this trend is related to the vast shortage of accredited internship positions in Canada, whose training is consistent with counselling psychology values, available for doctoral students (Haverkamp et al., 2011). Alternatively, counselling psychologists' presence in these non-traditional settings has the potential to bring about systemic change and alternative approaches in these settings (Haverkamp et al., 2011), although we are not aware of any research documenting that this is happening. Murkiness of professional identity, at the very least, puts counselling psychology at risk of being amalgamated into or at least integrated with a larger and more dominant overlapping profession, such as clinical psychology. This is already occurring as, recently, the University of Toronto switched its programme to offer a "Clinical and Counselling Psychology" doctoral programme. At the professional level, it could result in lower professional pride as differences from the predominant paradigm (e.g. less focus on diagnostic assessment, less emphasis on the medical model of working with individuals) could be seen as inferiorities and counselling psychologists may mimic higher status professionals doing similar work, such as clinical psychologists (see Beatch et al., 2009).

In terms of survey results operationalizing professional pride, respondents indicated that they were notably satisfied with their choice of counselling psychology as a career ($M = 5.2$, SD = 1.0, maximum value = 6) with 79.2% being "satisfied" or "very satisfied." Only one respondent (1.3%) was "very dissatisfied." However, when asked if they could go back and select a profession over again, only 48.0% stated that they would choose counselling psychology again while 26.7% stated that they would switch to clinical psychology, 6.7% to medicine, and 5.3% to each of law and counsellor education.

Conclusions

Counselling psychology in Canada has experienced tremendous growth and greater recognition within the last 30 years. The results of this study seem to imply that the majority of counselling psychologists in Canada are heterosexual women of European descent who were locally born and between 40 and 63 years of age. Most Canadian counselling psychologists are involved in providing privately paid psychological services to some extent. Of those who provide counselling or psychotherapy, it is usually of a rehabilitative-treatment nature and almost entirely with only a single individual at a time (vs. couples, family, or group counselling). Most Canadian counselling psychologists do not offer career counselling or vocational assessment (historical cornerstones of the profession) anymore and those who do only offer it for a small minority of their professional work-week. Overall, Canadian counselling psychologists seem to see the discipline as moderately differently from clinical psychology and counsellor education, and are satisfied with their choice of career in counselling psychology. However, although the majority of counselling psychologists in our study were satisfied or very satisfied with their career choice, only about 50% said that they would choose counselling psychology again as a career choice (with the most popular alternative being a career in clinical psychology). Lack of accredited internship sites espousing a counselling psychology orientation significantly cloud the development of professional identity as more counselling psychology students now intern at a medical facility rather than a counselling centre. Identity is also perhaps clouded by doctoral programmes accepting Master's students with education in fields other than counselling psychology.

The limitations of our survey are important to discuss. Many counselling psychologists in Canada are not members of the national psychology association (CPA) and the SCP. Unfortunately, there is no reliable estimate available of the total number of counselling psychologists in Canada or of the number who are not members of CPA and the SCP. It is highly possible that counselling psychologists who are not members of the SCP are different in some systematic ways (e.g. they may have higher rates of psychologist licensure or not be involved in research to the same extent). So although we can justifiably generalize our results to Canadian counselling psychologists who are members of the SCP, we can only speak cautiously about extending our results to the overall populace of Canadian counselling psychologists. In order to gain a more comprehensive understanding of the field and assess whether these results are truly representative of all Canadian counselling psychologists, future research should replicate this survey with counselling psychologists who are not members of the SCP. In addition, the predominance of respondents came from three of the thirteen provinces and territories (Alberta, Ontario and British Columbia) with no responses from Quebec which houses one of the five accredited training programmes. As such, results may only apply to those individuals working in English Canada and not apply to those working in Quebec or who identify as Francophone. Researchers should also administer this survey again in the future employing at least the same questions in order to track changes in the discipline in Canada over time.

Key articles

Key articles are noted in the references section with an asterisks. An updated list of significant readings is maintained by the SCP at http://www.cpa.ca/aboutcpa/cpasections/counsellingpsychology/readingsoncanadiancounselling

Disclosure statement

No potential conflict of interest was reported by the authors.

References

Recommended readings about Canadian counselling psychology are noted with an asterisk (*).

*Beatch, R., Bedi, R. P., Cave, D., Domene, J. F., Harris, G. E., Haverkamp, B. E., & Mikhail, A. (2009). *Counselling psychology in a Canadian context: Final report from the executive committee for a Canadian understanding of counselling psychology (report)*. Ottawa, ON: Counselling Psychology Section of the Canadian Psychological Association.

Bedi, R. P., & Domene, J. D. (2015). Canada: The case of Kamalpreet. In R. Moodley, M. Lengyell, R. Wu, & U.P Gielen (Eds.), *Therapy without borders: International and cross-cultural case studies* (pp. 141–148). Washington, DC: American Counseling Association.

*Bedi, R. P., Haverkamp, B. E., Beatch, R., Cave, D. G., Domene, J. F., Harris, G. E., & Mikhail, A. (2011). Counselling psychology in a Canadian context: Definition and description. *Canadian Psychology, 52*, 128–138.

*Bedi, R. P., Klubben, L. M., & Barker, G. T. (2012). Counselling vs. clinical: A comparison of psychology doctoral programs in Canada. *Canadian Psychology, 53*, 238–253.

Domene, J. D., & Bedi, R. P. (2013). Counseling and psychotherapy in Canada: Diversity and growth. In R. Moodley, U. P. Gielen, & R. Wu (Eds.), *Handbook of counseling and psychotherapy in an international context* (pp. 106–116). New York, NY: Routledge.

*Friesen, J. D. (1983). Counselling psychology: A discipline. *Canadian Counsellor, 17*, 147–154.

Goodyear, R. K., Lichtenberg, J. W., Hutman, H., Overland, E., Bedi, R., Christiani, K., ... Young, C. (in press). A global portrait of counselling psychologists' characteristics, perspectives, and professional behaviors. *Counselling Psychology Quarterly*. doi: 10.1080/09515070.2015.1128396

*Haverkamp, B. E., Robertson, S. R., Cairns, S. L., & Bedi, R. P. (2011). Professional issues in Canadian counseling psychology: Identity, education, and professional practice. *Canadian Psychology, 52*, 256–264.

*Hiebert, B., & Uhlemann, M. R. (1993). Counselling psychology: Development, identity, and issues. In K. S. Dobson & D. J. Dobson (Eds.), *Professional psychology in Canada* (pp. 286–312). Ashland, OH: Hogrefe & Huber.

Hurley, G. (2010). *Recollections of our past*. Keynote address presented at the Inaugural Canadian Counselling Psychology conference, Montreal, Quebec.

*Lalande, V. (2004). Counselling psychology: A Canadian perspective. *Counselling Psychology Quarterly, 17*, 273–286.

Linden, W., Moseley, J., & Erskine, Y. (2005). Psychology as a Health-Care Profession: Implications for training. *Canadian Psychology/Psychologie Canadienne, 46*, 179–188.

Linley, P. A. (2006). Counseling psychology's positive psychological agenda: A model for integration and inspiration. *The Counseling Psychologist, 34*, 313–322.

Schoenberg, B. M. (1988). *Annual report section on counselling*. Retrieved from http://cpa.ca/docs/File/Sections/Counselling/Annual%20Reports/AR_1986-87.pdf

Sinacore, A. L. (2015). Introduction. In A. L. Sinacore & F. Ginsberg (Eds.), *Canadian counselling and counselling psychology in the 21st century* (pp. 3–14). Montreal: McGill-Queens University Press.

*Sinacore, A. L., Borgen, W. A., Daniluk, J., Kassan, A., Long, B. C., & Nicol, J. J. (2011). Canadian counselling psychologists' contributions to applied psychology. *Canadian Psychology, 52*, 276–288.

*Young, R. A., & Lalande, V. (2011). Canadian counselling psychology: From defining moments to ways forward. *Canadian Psychology, 52*, 248–255.

*Young, R. A., & Nicol, J. J. (2007). Counselling psychology in Canada: Advancing psychology for all. *Applied Psychology: An International Review, 56*, 20–32.

Counselling psychology in New Zealand

Elizabeth du Preez[a], Jacqueline Feather[a] and Bill Farrell[b]

[a]Department of Psychology, Auckland University of Technology, Auckland, New Zealand;
[b]Private Practice, Titirangi, New Zealand

This article offers a brief overview of the history of counselling psychology in New Zealand. It describes current postgraduate study options and registration pathways as well as the institutions and organisations that provide legislative and professional membership and support to counselling psychologists in New Zealand. Data collected from a national survey in 2014 provide insight into the demographics of the profession in New Zealand, the theoretical frameworks that are utilised and employment opportunities that exist for counselling psychologists. The article also highlights the uniqueness of a cultural and contextual approach that aligns itself with New Zealand's founding document, the Treaty of Waitangi/te Tiriti o Waitangi which is based on the principles of partnership, participation and protection. It concludes with the challenges the profession face as a new scope of practice. These challenges include establishing a professional identity in the mental health delivery system in New Zealand and responding to an ever increasing multicultural society.

Counselling psychology (CP) is a relatively new and still-evolving paradigm in the landscape of psychology in Aotearoa[1]/New Zealand. As in other parts of the world, the informal roots of what has become CP have been present for many decades. In particular, key CP principles and practices in this country are inherent in the indigenous helping practices amongst New Zealand's first people, the Māori (Farrell, 2013). However, the formal history of CP in New Zealand began when the professional body for counselling psychologists, the New Zealand Psychological Society's (NZPsS) Institute of Counselling Psychology (ICounsPsy), was formed in September 2003, as a successor to the Society's former *Counselling* Division.

New Zealand's first (and, so far, only) training in CP, at Auckland University of Technology (AUT), admitted its first students in 2006. An application to the New Zealand Psychologists Board, the government regulator of the professional practice of psychology, for a Counselling Psychologist Scope of Practice was approved in 2010, and the AUT programme received Psychologists Board Accreditation for training in CP in 2011. In 2014, the Psychologists Board approved specific competencies for the CP scope of practice under the Health Practitioners Competence Assurance Act (Ministry of Health, 2003). This act regulates health professionals in New Zealand, including counselling psychologists (New Zealand Psychologists Board, 2012). This scope of practice now forms a benchmark, spelling out what it means to be a registered counselling psychologist in New Zealand.

Counselling psychologists in New Zealand

Counselling psychologists in New Zealand are broadly made up of three groups: "grand-parents," including those who were practicing as counselling psychologists before accredited training and registration were available; graduates and current students from the AUT programme; and, counselling psychologists who trained overseas and have had their training and qualifications recognised by the Psychologists Board.

This diversity is reflected in the national survey we conducted, some of which is reported in Goodyear et al. (in press). In particular, only 47% ($N = 24$) of the participants held a degree in CP, whilst the rest indicated that they had received training in the areas of clinical psychology, counselling, marriage and family therapy, educational and community psychology, health psychology, or vocational guidance and counselling. Whereas three-fourths (76%) of the participants' degrees were accredited by the New Zealand Psychologists Board, all but two of the remaining 24 had qualifications that were not accredited by any other professional association either.

Training and registration as a counselling psychologist in New Zealand

The New Zealand Psychologists Board (2012) specifies the following requirements for registration as a counselling psychologist:

> … a minimum of a Master's degree in psychology from an accredited educational organisation and an accredited Postgraduate Diploma in Counselling psychology, or equivalent qualification. Eligibility for a Counselling Psychologist scope of practice shall require a Board approved practicum or internship involving 1500 h of supervised practice.

The Psychologists Board has also agreed to a period of "grand-parenting" into the Counselling Psychologist Scope of Practice, which will be available until 31 March 2016. This enables the founders of the practice tradition in New Zealand to gain recognition for their portfolios of qualification which were gained when formal professional training was not available as equivalent to that which leads to registration as a counselling psychologist.

The AUT counselling psychology programme includes a Bachelor of Health Science Honours degree as well as the successful application for and completion of a Master's in Health Science in Psychology and a Postgraduate Diploma in Counselling Psychology. The Postgraduate Diploma consists of a 1500-h supervised internship as well as coursework requirements as specified by the university and accredited by the New Zealand Psychologists Board. The training, like CP internationally, positions itself as a union between scientific models of functioning and more humanistic, contextual views (Scherman & Feather, 2013). Frameworks for practice include empowerment/enhancement, phenomenological, developmental, systemic, cultural, ethical and spiritual. The intervention models taught include systemic, cognitive behavioural and third-wave therapies such as

Acceptance and Commitment Therapy. Of interest is that whereas the most frequently endorsed theoretical model was cognitive behavioural (27.8% of New Zealand participants; Table 7; Goodyear et al., in press), 39.7% endorsed an eclectic or integrationist perspective, with a few participants then indicating that they practice from a wide variety of other theoretical orientations.

The place of CP in the health delivery system in New Zealand

Health services in New Zealand are delivered by several organisations that sit within the portfolio of the Minister of Health. The day-to-day delivery of services is administered by 20 District Health Boards (DHB's) and Health Workforce New Zealand advises the Ministry of Health on employment matters, including the identification of health practitioners who are deemed appropriate for roles in the DHB's (Ministry of Health, 2014). CP is currently not on the list of scopes included on the government funded careers website (www.careers.govt.nz) and DHB's employ mainly clinical psychologists, and sometimes, depending on their needs, child psychotherapists, especially in Child and Adolescent Mental Health Services. Students and graduates from the CP programme at AUT have obtained internships and employment primarily in Non-Government Funded Organisations (NGOs) and university settings. Examples include mental health rehabilitation services, alcohol, drug and problem gambling agencies, physical health settings such as the Cancer Society, hospice services, integrated health clinics, primary health care organisations, family based intervention services and university student counselling and community clinics.

Two-thirds of the survey participants indicated that they predominantly work in private practice settings and NGOs (which were coded as "other" in Table 3, Goodyear et al., in press) while the remainder work in university counselling centres, psychology departments and 1% of survey respondents indicated that they were employed in a hospital setting. All of the respondents indicated that they were satisfied with their careers as counselling psychologists, with 90% of participants reporting being satisfied or very satisfied with their choice of career.

Professional CP organisations

The only professional association in New Zealand exclusively for counselling psychologists is the Institute of Counselling Psychology, a part of the New Zealand Psychological Society (NZPsS). Virtually all (98%) of the survey participants were members of the Society. Although only 32% said they held student memberships during their studies, we are aware this has increased recently with better links between NZPsS and training programmes.

The other major organisation for psychologists is the New Zealand College of Clinical Psychologists (NZCCP), formed exclusively for clinical psychologists by some of their members who moved away from the NZPsS in the late 1980s (New Zealand College of Clinical Psychologists, 2015). Because of NZCCP's exclusive focus on clinical psychology, counselling psychologists are not eligible to join.

Counselling psychology in relation to other specialties and professions

A key relationship for CP, in New Zealand as elsewhere, is that with clinical psychology. In 2004, Gibson and colleagues (Gibson, Stanley, & Manthei, 2004) described CP as a practice and how it could possibly contribute to psychological service delivery in New Zealand. This was published in the NZPsS *Bulletin*, (the regular publication for the profession, subsequently renamed *Psychology Aotearoa*) and met by an initial response of resistance in the subsequent issue from Fitzgerald and colleagues (Fitzgerald, Calvert, Thorburn, Collie, & Marsh, 2005) that could hardly be seen as welcoming. In the decade since, CP's relationship with clinical psychology has continued to develop and remains a potential focus for cooperation as well as challenge and tension. Of note is that a Special Section of the *New Zealand Journal of Psychology* on CP was published in 2013. In this section, Scherman and Feather (2013) identified the struggle for CP identity locally as a theme common to CP internationally (Scherman & Feather, 2013).

Another key relationship is between CP and the profession of psychotherapy, which is the more established profession in New Zealand. The New Zealand Association of Psychotherapists was founded in 1948, with formal professional training becoming available in 1986, and psychotherapist registration in 2007. A number of New Zealand CPs are also trained and experienced psychotherapists, but the registration system that has been adopted focuses on title protection, so only Registered Psychotherapists can call themselves a "psychotherapist." If counselling psychologists who are also psychotherapists wish to claim that title, they are required to obtain *and maintain* a second registration, which is a considerable expense in a country with a small population. The only university-based psychotherapy training in New Zealand is in the same Faculty at AUT as the CP programme, and there is some overlap in the curriculum. But as yet there are few formal links between the professions.

Traditions and core values that are definitive of New Zealand CP

CP in New Zealand is shaped not only by the professional values that are unique to CP as a psychology specialty, but also by its commitment to the principles inherent in the Treaty of Waitangi/*te Tiriti o Waitangi* (1840), New Zealand's founding document. An agreement for partnership between the indigenous Māori and the European settlers that was signed in 1840 by Māori chiefs and the British Crown, the Treaty continues to be a "living document" that provides guidance for our bicultural nation. It embodies the principles of *partnership, participation* and *active protection* which strongly influence health policy and delivery (National Advisory Committee on Health and Disability, 2002), including that of psychology.

The Code of Ethics for Psychologists Working in Aotearoa/New Zealand (2002) outlines four Principles: Respect for the dignity of persons and peoples, responsible caring, integrity in relationships, and social justice and responsibility to society. These include non-discrimination, sensitivity to diversity, as well as explicit responsibility for psychologists to recognise that the Treaty of Waitangi sets out the basis of respect between Māori and non- Māori in this country. In addition, the New Zealand Psychologists Board has developed Standards of Cultural Competence (2011) for psychologists registered under the Health Practitioners Competence Assurance Act (2003) and those seeking to become registered. This is a framework that reflects cultural safety, the

Treaty of Waitangi, and international cultural competence standards. Of course, New Zealand is now a highly sophisticated and cosmopolitan society with people of many nations and cultural and ethnic backgrounds who have settled here since the early British settlers. However, the Treaty and the bicultural practice models that emanated from it continue to be a template for providing for the needs of this increasingly population.

The New Zealand Psychological Society (NZPsS) has adopted the following definition of CP that reflect the core values and approaches to well-being:

> (Counselling psychology is) a psychological specialty that utilises and applies psychological knowledge and research at the individual, group and organisational level. Counselling psychologists enable and empower clients experiencing typical and atypical problems of living to enhance their personal, social, educational and vocational functioning.
>
> The specialty embraces a range of approaches including preventative and educational programmes, and acknowledges the importance of phenomenological perspectives as well as the influence of developmental and ecological factors.

This definition also adds:

> The Institute (of Counselling Psychology) is established with a commitment to biculturalism and cultural diversity, in the interests of the public and the profession, to promote the highest standards of knowledge and practice in counselling psychology in Aotearoa/New Zealand. (New Zealand Psychological Society, 2012)

In the survey (see Goodyear et al., in press), New Zealand participants endorsed core values that were largely consistent with this definition.

Major issues and opportunities for CP in New Zealand

New Zealand CP has a relatively short local history that started in 2003 with the formation of the NZPsS Institute of Counselling Psychology. With this newness comes both challenges and opportunities as CPs align themselves with the core values of not only the profession but also to the particular contextual demands of New Zealand society.

New Zealand is increasingly regarded as a multicultural country with the 2013 New Zealand census identifying 213 ethnic groups. New Zealand European, Māori, Chinese, Samoan and Indian are the five largest ethnic groups and since the 2006 census the biggest increase has occurred within the Chinese, Indian and Filipino ethnic groups. Over the last seven years the Middle Eastern/Latin American/African and Asian ethnic groups have also increased by more than 30% (Statistics New Zealand, 2013).

Working in partnership with Māori, and across multiple cultures continues to be both a challenge and opportunity as the major professional organisations and the New Zealand Psychologists Board embraces its commitment to the Treaty of Waitangi and the principles of a bicultural relationship based on partnership, participation and protection. Counselling psychology in New Zealand views cultural competence as an ethical practice issue as described in the Cultural Competencies Document (New Zealand Psychologists Board, 2006). It emphasizes contextual understanding and encourages working from models of practice based on a Māori world view, as well as models from all cultures represented in New Zealand, where appropriate.

Another challenge for CPs is gaining employment in the New Zealand job market. As mentioned earlier, CP is not included in Health Workforce New Zealand (Ministry of Health, 2015) scopes of practice, and counselling psychologists are therefore generally not considered for employment in District Health Board positions. The advantage of this is that CP has been given an opportunity to develop a strong professional identity which is not associated with a particular employment role. Nevertheless, the lack of government investment and community knowledge results in fewer employment opportunities and lower income prospects with NGO-funded roles (Farrell, 2013). In response to open-ended questions about challenges they perceived, survey respondents raised this as a significant issue and consider this an area in which the Institute of Counselling Psychology could support their members in more effective ways.

Sir James Henare's words, as included in the foreword to the Te Tai Tokerau Māori Health Strategic Plan 2008–2013 (Northland District Health Board, 2013) also resonates when thinking about the future of CP in New Zealand:

> Kua tawhiti ke to haerenga mai, kia kore e haere tonu. He tino nui rawa ou mahi, kia kore e mahi nui tonu.

> You have come too far, not to go further. You have done too much, not to do more. (Ta Himi Henare Ngati Hine, 1989)

Counselling psychology is a developing paradigm in New Zealand which is grounded in a privileging of the therapeutic relationship (Milton, 2011) within a culturally appropriate and collaborative framework. As a relatively young scope of practice in New Zealand, it will continue to explore ways of contributing to the mental health and well-being of the growing and increasingly diverse population residing in this country.

Key articles and resources

Evans, I. M., Rucklidge, J. J., & O'Driscoll, M. (Eds.). (2007). *Professional practice of psychology in Aotearoa New Zealand*. Wellington: New Zealand Psychological Society.

Taylor, A. J. W. (1997). Collegiate psychology in New Zealand: The early days of the Society. *Bulletin of the New Zealand Psychological Society, 92*, 14–17.

Disclosure statement

No potential conflict of interest was reported by the authors.

Note

1. Aotearoa is the Māori name for New Zealand. Māori are the indigenous people and it is out of respect that we refer to the Māori name for our country, however it is not the official name so we will use New Zealand throughout the remainder of the article.

References

Farrell, W. B. F. (2013). Counselling psychology in Aotearoa/New Zealand: What is it, where has it come from, and where might it go? *New Zealand Journal of Psychology, 42*, 11–17.

Fitzgerald, J., Calvert, S., Thorburn, J., Collie, R., & Marsh, J. (2005). Counselling psychology in New Zealand and the use of bi-focal lenses: A reply to Gibson, Stanley and Manthei's article. *The Bulletin of the New Zealand Psychological Society, 104*, 23–25.

Gibson, K., Stanley, P., & Manthei, R. (2004). Counselling psychology in New Zealand: A window of opportunity. *The Bulletin of the New Zealand Psychological Society, 103*, 12–17.

Goodyear, R. K., Lichtenberg, J. W., Hutman, H., Overland, E., Bedi, R., Christiani, K., … Young, C. (in press). A global portrait of counselling psychologists' characteristics, perspectives, and professional behaviors. *Counselling Psychology Quarterly.* doi: 10.1080/09515070.2015.1128396

Milton, M. (2011, August). *Holding the tension: Relational perspectives in counselling psychology practice.* Keynote presented at the New Zealand Psychological Society Annual Conference, Queenstown, New Zealand.

Ministry of Health. (2003). Health Practitioners Competence Assurance Act. Retrieved March 5, 2015, from http://www.health.govt.nz/our-work/regulation-health-and-disability-system/health-practitioners-competence-assurance-act

Ministry of Health. (2014). District Health Boards. Retrieved March 5, 2015, from http://www.health.govt.nz/new-zealand-health-system/key-health-sector-organisations-and-people/district-health-boards

Ministry of Health. (2015). Health Workforce. Retrieved March 3, from http://www.health.govt.nz/our-work/health-workforce

National Advisory Commitee on Health and Disability (2002). Eleventh Annual Report to the Minister of Health. Retrieved December 23, 2015 from https://nhc.health.govt.nz/system/files/documents/publications/nhc-annual-report-2002.pdf

New Zealand College of Clinical Psychologists. (2015). Retrieved February 12, 2015, from http://www.nzccp.co.nz

New Zealand Psychological Society. (2012). *The Institute of Counselling psychology.* Retrieved December 23, 2015, from http://www.psychology.org.nz/membership/member-groups/institute-of-counselling-psychology/#.VnjNNBV97IV

New Zealand Psychologists Board. (2006). *Cultural competencies.* Wellington: New Zealand-Psychologists Board.

New Zealand Psychologists Board. (2012). Developing Core Competencies for the Counselling Psychologist Scope: Initial Consultation and Call for Nominations. Retrieved July 14, 2012, from http://www.psychologistsboard.org.nz/cms_show_download.php?id=178

Northland District Health Board. (2013). Te Tai Tokerau Maori Health Strategic Plan 2008-2013. Retrieved March 5, 2015, from http://www.northlanddhb.org.nz/Portals/0/Communications/Publications/ttt%20maori%20strategic%20plan%20final.pdf

Scherman, R. M., & Feather, J. S. (2013). Counselling psychology in Aotearoa/New Zealand: Introduction to the special section. *New Zealand Journal of Psychology, 42*, 7–10.

Statistics New Zealand. (2013). 2013 Census ethnic group profiles. Retrieved March 7, 2015, from http://www.stats.govt.nz/Census/2013-census/profile-and-summary-reports/ethnic-profiles.aspx

Counselling psychology in South Africa

Jason Bantjes[a], Ashraf Kagee[a] and Charles Young[b]

[a]Department of Psychology, Stellenbosch University, Stellenbosch, South Africa; [b]Psychology Department, Rhodes University, Grahamstown, South Africa

The origin and development of counselling psychology in South Africa has been profoundly influenced by the country's sociopolitical history and the impact of apartheid. As a result of this, counselling psychologists in the country face a number of challenges and opportunities for the future. In this paper we provide a portrait of counselling psychology in South Africa by describing the current character of the specialty and the context in which South African psychologists work. We critically discuss the challenges that the specialty faces to meet the country's mental health care needs, contest the current Scope of Practice; affirm multiculturalism without essentialising or reifying race and ethnicity, and build an evidence base for community interventions in the country. We also consider how, in the future, counselling psychologists in South Africa may make a more meaningful contribution within public health and the country's health care and education systems.

Counselling psychology (CP) in South Africa (SA) has a fairly brief and exclusionary history and many of the challenges the specialty faces reflect the country's colonial past and the sociopolitical and economic consequences of apartheid. Despite a four-decade history, CP in post-apartheid SA has yet to achieve a recognisable, coherent and socially relevant professional identity that differentiates the speciality from the other branches of applied psychology (Leach, Akhurst, & Basson, 2003; Watson & Fouche, 2007; Young, 2013). In this paper, we briefly describe the origins of the specialty in SA. We consider the current character of CP, describe the contemporary context in which SA counselling psychologists (CPs) practice and discuss the challenges faced by the profession.

A brief history of counselling psychology in SA

Among the several accounts of South African CP development (Leach et al., 2003; Painter & Terre Blanche, 2004; Van Ommen & Painter, 2008), the one by Leach et al., provides a particular challenge to the specialty. Leach et al. (2003) trace the origin of CP to Stellenbosch University, an Afrikaans-language tertiary institution, which is considered to be the intellectual cradle of Afrikaner nationalism and which had appointed H. F. Verwoerd (one of the major architects of apartheid) as professor of applied psychology in 1927. They assert that, CP was set up in opposition to clinical psychology and was primarily concerned with serving the goals of the nationalist government, addressing the career development and psychological well-being of the minority White Afrikaans-speaking citizens (Cooper, Nicholas, Seedat, & Statman, 1990; Foster, 1993; Leach et al., 2003). This focus on vocational issues and health promotion mirrors the evolution of the CP in the US (Cook & Visser, 1986). However, unlike in the US, the new discipline of CP in SA sought explicitly to uplift economically marginalised Whites in order to retain economic power in the hands of the White minority (Leach et al., 2003). Although this emphasis is no longer true, it is a legacy that CP has worked to overcome in SA.

The professional category of "Counselling Psychologist" was not recognised in SA until 1974 (Government Gazette, 1974), at which time professional training programmes were established at four Afrikaans-speaking universities (Stellenbosch, Port Elizabeth, Bloemfontein, and Rand Afrikaans) and at one English-speaking university (The University of Natal, Pietermaritzburg; Leach et al., 2003), all of which were at the time only accessible to White students. As a result, the specialty initially was dominated by White, Afrikaans-speaking men. More recently professional training programmes have been initiated at a number of English-speaking universities and at universities which were previously reserved for Black students. Today, CP programmes are located at English- and Afrikaans-language universities, and historically-white and historically-black universities. In total, 13 institutions are accredited to offer postgraduate CP training (though two of these programmes are currently in abeyance) (Daffue, personal communication, 2014).

Credentialing of counselling psychologists in SA

To practice as a counselling psychologist in SA it is necessary to register with the Health Professions Council of SA (HPCSA). Prerequisites for registration are successful completion of a four-year degree in psychology, an accredited master's degree in CP (1 year), a one-year internship, and successful completion of the Board Examination (HPCSA, 2013a). While clinical psychologists and other members of the medical and allied health professions, are required to complete a compulsory year of community service before they may practice independently, there is no such requirement for CPs.

The place of counselling psychology in SA's health system

SA is a country characterised by high rates of mental disorders and inadequate mental health care services (Herman et al., 2009). Health care services are also unequally distributed within the country and are delivered via a government funded public health care system (which serves the majority of the country's citizens) and a private health care system (which serves the comparatively small group of wealthy people).

At present the state mental health system only has posts for clinical psychologists, although this was not always the case. In 1996 the number of CPs in full-time state employment was significantly larger than the number of clinical psychologists and approximately 17% of the country's CPs were employed in the public service (Pillay & Petersen, 1996). The most recent SA survey, conducted in 2014 (see Goodyear et al., in press) suggests that this proportion may now be as little as 4%.

The limited employment opportunities for CPs in the country's public health care system has resulted in a decline in the popularity of counselling training programmes, with many masters students instead electing training in clinical psychology to improve their employment opportunities. Some universities (e.g. Stellenbosch University and the University of the Western Cape) have discontinued their counselling masters programmes partly as a result of this trend. Towards the end of 2014, there were 1661 counselling psychologists registered with the Health Professions Council, which constituted 21% of all registered psychologists (Daffue, personal communication, 2014). This represented a decline from 2002 when CPs constituted approximately 35% of all registered psychologists (Leach et al., 2003).

A senior official in the national Department of Health has indicated the need for a change so that CPs may find employment in the public health system (Freeman, personal communication, 8 December 2014). We argue that CPs can be effectively used within clinical settings at the interface of medicine, psychiatry and psychology. In this context, the absence of formal training and practice opportunities in health psychology in SA is significant. We believe that, in keeping with many other parts of the world, CPs in SA as practitioners of health psychology have a role to play in general medical settings, for example, in helping patients with issues such as adherence to treatment, management of chronic illness, diseases of lifestyle, pain-management, the psychological issues associated with disability and family functioning in the context of disability and chronic illness.

In spite of the lack of CP posts within the public health care system, CPs in SA can be found in a variety of public and private sectors, including the police services, military, universities, schools, NGOs, community organisations, social service organisations and industry (Watson & Fouche, 2007). Yet, recent data show that the range of employment options for CPs outside of private practice and higher education are limited. Currently, almost half of all CPs (48.9%) work in private practice, a setting that excludes the economically marginalised mostly black residents of the country. Another third are employed by universities (13.6% at university counselling centres; 15.8% at university psychology departments; and 3.2% in other university departments) (reference to survey). The results of such limited employment opportunities outside of private practice is that many CPs must adopt an entrepreneurial rather than an altruistic approach to their work, an emphasis that does not fit very well with the values of CP (Packard, 2009; Young, 2013).

Another factor that has contributed to inaccessibility of services is that most CPs in the country do not speak the indigenous languages of the Black majority (de la Rey & Ipser, 2004; Watson & Fouche, 2007). This reality has contributed to the significant treatment gap that exists in the country and remains a challenge for contemporary CPs.

Professional organisations in SA

The statutory registration of psychologists is governed by the Health Professions Council of SA (HPCSA), a body that comprises 12 Professional Boards, one of which is the Professional Board for Psychology (Health Professions Act 56, 1974). The Professional Board for Psychology recognises clinical, counselling, research, industrial, educational, forensic and neuro-psychology as separate categories of registration and mandates separate scopes of practice for each (Government Gazette, 2011). The HPCSA has also made provision for the registration of professional counsellors (who have completed 4 years of university training) to practice in a limited capacity offering counselling services. Professional counsellors are mandated to provide screening and basic psychological interventions as the first line of community based psychological support.

Professional psychology in SA is organised by the Psychological Society of SA (PsySSA), which was established in 1994, the same year in which SA had its first democratic elections. The organisation has 13 divisions of which the Association for CP is one. PsySSA publishes the country's only general-interest psychology journal, the *South African Journal of Psychology* (SAJP), and hosts the annual South African Psychology Congress (Cooper, 2014). Unlike the HPCSA, membership of the organisation is voluntary.

Counselling psychology's relationship to clinical psychology and other health care workers

While CP in SA is considered to be distinct from clinical psychology, the two subfields have considerable overlap In fact, several training institutions combine clinical and counselling training, which serves to further diffuse differences between the two subfields.

In 2011 a new scope of practice (SoP) for the Psychology Profession was promulgated into law in SA (Government Gazette, 2011). The SoP has sought to redefine overlapping but essentially separate scopes of practice for clinical and CP. Within this framework clinical psychologists are restricted to work that entails "identifying psychopathology in psychiatric disorders and psychological conditions" (Government Gazette, 2011, p. 6) and "identifying, and diagnosing psychiatric disorders and psychological conditions" (Government Gazette, 2011, p. 6). The work of CPs, on the other hand, is delineated as "assessing, diagnosing, and intervening in clients dealing with life challenges, and developmental problems to optimise psychological wellbeing" (Government Gazette, 2011, p. 7) and "assessing cognitive, personality, emotional and neuropsychological functions in relation to life challenges and developmental problems" (Government Gazette, 2011, p. 7). The SoP thus makes a distinction between *psychopathology* and *life challenges/wellbeing/adjustment*. It states explicitly that psychopathology is the domain of clinical psychologists and that CPs are concerned only with health development, as if these two domains are distinct and easily differentiated. Explicit in the new SoP is the directive that clinical psychologists focus on "treating psychological and psychiatric conditions", (Government Gazette, 2011, p. 6) and CPs focus on "offering counselling interventions to resolve development issues and adjustment disorders" (Government Gazette, 2011, p. 7). Though the practical implications of the SoP remain unclear, some practitioners have already interpreted the SoP very narrowly to mean that CPs should not intervene to remediate psychopathology (Botha, 2011). The training and practice of counselling and clinical psychology in SA have always overlapped considerably (Leach et al., 2003; Pillay & Petersen, 1996). As such, many CPs, especially the large proportion who earn their living by offering psychotherapy in private practice, are wary of any revisions to their SoP that might curtail aspects of their professional work and negate part of their experience and training. The wording of the SoP explicitly focuses CP on so-called "life challenges" and "adjustment and developmental problems". A narrow interpretation of the SoP implies that the practice of CP in SA is inextricably tied up with: "typical problems of living" (Government

Gazette, 2011). These problems include educational problems, relationship difficulties, divorce, bereavement, crime, accidents, substance use, retirement, unemployment, physical illness and disability. However, they may also more broadly refer to social problems such as poverty, unemployment and social inequality (Seekings & Nattrass, 2006); gender-based (Abrahams et al., 2009) and other forms of interpersonal violence (Kaminer, Grimsrud, Myer, Stein, & Williams, 2008); and an HIV prevalence that is amongst the highest in the world (Department of Health, 2012), occurring in a context of severe HIV stigma (Kalichman et al., 2005). Furthermore a broad interpretation of *life challenges, adjustment and developmental problems* arguably also includes many of the mild-to-moderate anxiety, eating, substance abuse, trauma and depressive disorders that are typically borne by people who continue to meet, for the most part, their social and occupational obligations. This broad reading of the SoP is consistent with the various international definitions of CP (Pelling, 2004; Young, 2013).

The source of much of the confusion about the SoP of CP is related to its traditional emphasis on people's strengths. Yet, as Bedi et al. (2011, p. 131) argue, a "[f]ocus on strengths does not imply a particular scope of practice; rather, it represents an instance where the field's philosophical orientation infuses multiple areas of its practice." Thus while developmental work is considered a defining feature of CP (Savickas, 2007), surveys in the USA have revealed that, as the discipline has matured, there has been a gradual shift in the practice of CPs towards clinical remediation (Goodyear et al., 2008). While CPs in SA have an important role to play in remediating psychopathology, this need not be at the expense of prevention and development (Young, 2013).

Major issues, opportunities and threats for counselling psychology in SA

By virtue of SA's history and the country's current sociocultural and mental health care context, CP faces a number of challenges. These include finding ways to overcome apartheid's legacy of inequality and engage critically with the call to advance a social justice agenda and work as agents of change while embracing the evidence-based practice movement. The specialty also needs to achieve greater racial diversity, make a meaningful contribution to meeting the country's mental health care needs, apply psychological knowledge to promote physical health and well-being and respond to the call to indigenise the practice of psychology. Each of these challenges is described and critically discussed below.

Overcoming apartheid's legacy of inequality and adopting a social justice agenda

SA continues to grapple with the enduring legacy of apartheid, a system of oppressive educational, economic, social, political and geographical measures that deprived the majority of black South Africans from full citizenship, adequate social services, skills and life opportunities, in order to sustain white economic privilege. Despite the transition to democratic rule in 1994, deep inequalities remain a feature of SA society. The challenge to CPs is to adopt the agenda of community psychology and find a way to utilise their skills and knowledge to promote economic liberation in SA and disrupt current social structures that maintain inequality.

In the last decade, SA's CPs increasingly have come under fire for failing to be relevant and to practise their specialty in a socially responsible way. Leach et al. (2003)

maintain that CPs need to prove their viability to other professions and the community at large by addressing the social ills currently facing the country. Critics have also noted the specialty's need to adopt an increasingly greater advocacy role (Foster, 2004) and play a more proactive role in addressing educational, social, racial and gender issues (de la Rey & Ipser, 2004). It has been suggested that CPs need to extend their reach and adopt advocacy roles; engage in community interventions; become integrally involved in policy formation and actively change social structures (Vera & Speight, 2003; Young, 1990).

Counselling psychology and cultural relevance

Critics have called attention to CP's Euro-American bias (Painter & Terre Blanche, 2004) and its propensity to employ theoretical models developed for wealthy White Western individuals. CPs have thus been prompted to engage actively with the indigenisation of counselling theory and practice in SA (Stead & Watson, 2006), which is in keeping with multiculturalism as a "fourth force" in psychological practice. Given the historical bias of CP towards Euro-American psychological theories and models, as well as the lack of access of most Black South Africans to psychological services, it is incumbent on contemporary SA CPs to imagine ways in which the specialty may be indigenised. While we acknowledge the need for culturally sensitive psychological interventions, we caution against an essentialising view of culture that seeks to construct non-Western cultural practices as exotic and mysterious; such practices create a false dichotomy by constructing "African" and "Western" cultural contexts and systems of healing as discrete entities. Globalisation has seen to it that many countries in the global South, including SA, probably share more cultural currency with the global North than is usually considered. It is more likely that Southern African countries, including SA, occupy a hybrid cultural space that straddles "Western" and African cultures. In such a context, hybrid psychological interventions may be well placed as long as they provide measurable benefit to help seekers. Many African countries, including SA, are characterised by concerns such as migration, urbanisation, township and suburban life, social media and its attendant deluge of information. To this extent, a single monolithic African culture does not exist and it is necessary for CP to make itself relevant to this culturally complex context.

The evidence to date is encouraging and suggests that models developed in Western contexts may be effectively adapted and applied in a variety of African settings (e.g. Bolton et al., 2003, 2007; Igreja, Kleijn, Schreuder, van Dijk, & Verschuur, 2004; Neuner et al., 2008). The challenge for CP in SA is thus to integrate its essential principles of multiculturalism with an acknowledgement of the multicultural and multiethnic character of the country without essentialising and reifying race and ethnicity.

Building an evidence-base for community interventions

Community psychology is a well-developed subdiscipline in SA and overlaps with CP and is an integral component of professional CP training. Community psychology interventions in SA as well as other sub-Saharan African countries place a focus on topical issues such as school bullying, youth at risk for crime, teenage pregnancy, safer sex, anti-violence programmes and parenting skills. While empirical evidence for these interventions may not always exist, we take the view that psychologists-in-training should be exposed to treatment protocols informed by the best available evidence if the interventions they apply in community settings are to be optimally effective. The implicit challenge to CPs in SA is to contribute to establishing a body of knowledge and evidence to support their community interventions.

Counselling psychology and the evidence-based movement

A significant anomaly is apparent in the new scope of practice in that clinical psychologists are explicitly required to offer evidence-based interventions, while no such prescription is incumbent on CP. The wording of the current SoP and the important omission of references to interventions which are evidence-based is important and reflects a greater problem in the practice of professional psychology in SA. The evidence-based movement in psychology seeks to promote effective psychological practice in the service of contributing to public health. It does so by adhering to empirically supported principles in the context of psychological assessment, formulation of individual cases, establishing the therapeutic relationship, and implementing psychological interventions (American Psychological Association, 2015). Adhering to evidence-based practice in SA is an important issue, especially given the limited mental health care resources and the need to ensure that interventions are effective.

Kagee (2006) has argued that this notable absence may be in part due to the nature of clinical and CP training programmes that themselves place an inordinate emphasis on poorly validated therapeutic procedures while overvaluing clinical intuition.

Achieving greater diversity within the specialty

SA, a country with a population of approximately 53 million (The World Bank, 2015), is served by 10,961 registered psychologists and 799 psychiatrists (HPCSA, 2013b). Table 1 below shows the racial and gender distribution of psychologists by categories of registration as on 2 February 2015 (HPCSA, private communication). It is apparent from Table 1 that although a gender transformation has occurred as a result of the feminisation of the specialty, the racial profile still fails to reflect the country's racial and language demographics. There is a clear need for transformation and diversification of the specialty within the country.

Meeting the mental health care needs of the country

SA has a high prevalence of mental disorders but inadequate mental health care. A survey of a nationally representative cohort of adults found that 30.3% of the sample reported having a mental disorder at some point in their lives, (Herman et al., 2009). Evidence indicates that 15.9% of people living in SA had received some form of medical or psychological treatment in the past 12 months, while only 25.2% of individuals with a mental disorder had sought treatment within the general medical sector, and only 5.7% had received care from a mental health care professional (Seedat et al., 2009). These findings suggest that a large number of South Africans experience symptoms of psychological distress but that there is a substantial treatment gap with very few receiving the care they need. A lack of resources is not the only factor that restricts access to

Table 1. Racial and gender profile of registered psychologists in South Africa by category of registration (as on 2 February 2015).

	Race	Female	Male	Total
Clinical psychology (including community service clinical psychologists)	African	367	120	487
	Coloured	82	27	109
	Indian	127	27	154
	Not known	356	235	591
	White	1155	469	1624
Total number of clinical psychologists		2087	878	2965
Counselling psychology	African	115	38	153
	Coloured	52	16	68
	Indian	81	19	100
	Not known	208	109	317
	White	762	252	1014
Total number of counselling psychology		1218	434	1652

mental health care in SA. Cultural barriers, including stigma associated with seeking mental health services, also reduce the likelihood of people receiving the treatment they need.

Given the high rates of mental disorders and the significant lack of access to mental health care services, there is an implicit challenge to CPs in SA to apply their knowledge and skill in order to help close this treatment gap. In the context of the small number of CPs in many LMIC's, one option for the provision of comparable services is the deployment of non-specialists such as primary health care staff including nurses, nursing assistants, professional counsellors, as well as lay community health workers. Such professionals and para-professionals may provide a range of services such as screening, assessment, counselling, and evaluation of symptoms of common mental disorders and problems in living. The challenge to CPs will be to find a way to support this task shifting and provide on-going supervision and training of those tasked with providing mental health care.

Making a contribution to the promotion of health

Many SA communities are characterised by high rates of communicable diseases such as HIV and tuberculosis as well as non-communicable diseases such as diabetes, hypertension and heart disease. SA has for many years been the country with the largest number of persons living with HIV and AIDS (PLWHA). PLWHA have an elevated risk of being diagnosed with a mental disorder compared to the general population (Freeman, Nkomo, Kafaar, & Kelly, 2008; Olley, Seedat, Nei, & Stein, 2004). In addition, common mental disorders are associated with a lower likelihood of receiving antiretroviral treatment (ART) (Turner, Laine, Cosler, & Hauck, 2003) and lower rates of adherence to ART (Ammassari et al., 2002; Catz, Kelly, Bogart, Benotsch, & McAuliffe, 2000; Spire et al., 2002). However, the integration of mental health interventions into HIV/AIDS care and treatment in most developing countries has been slow (Freeman, Patel, Collins, & Bertolote, 2005). In SA, providing psychological support and patient advocacy has been taken up mainly by counsellors and lay persons who have rudimentary counselling training. The need thus exists for CPs to avail themselves to fulfil this important role.

Responding to the mental health needs of immigrants and refugees

By definition, a refugee is one who has been forced to flee their homeland because of fear of persecution on the basis of race, religion, nationality, or membership of a social or political group (UNHCR, 1951). Flight from one country to another is premised on some or other form of physical danger, which in many instances may include the psychological experience of traumatisation or at least some form of psychological distress. Refugee flight may also be accompanied by temporary or permanent loss of family members such as children or parents, loss of material belongings including one's home, the legal and logistical challenges of obtaining refugee status in another country as well as the practical challenges of making a life in a new environment. Various estimates indicate that SA may have as many as five million undocumented immigrants (Minaar, Pretorius, & Wentzel, 1995), with at least three million from Zimbabwe.

In addition to the severe stresses of migration, in 2008 and 2015 SA witnessed a wave of xenophobic violence against foreign nationals, many of whom were economic migrants, asylum seekers and refugees. Such challenges create specific and unique mental health needs that may be uniquely within the ambit of CP to address. If the mandate of CPs is to address problems in living among members of the general population rather than those of psychiatric patients, then the needs of refugees and displaced persons fall within this remit.

Key articles

Watson and Fouche (2007) note that while much has been written about professional psychology in SA, very little of this is specifically about the practice of CP. Only three articles that specifically deal with CP in SA have been published since the new millennium; namely Leach et al. (2003); Watson and Fouche (2007) and Young (2013). While Leach et al. (2003) and Watson and Fouche (2007) provide critical discussions of the history and inadequacies of CP in SA, Young's (2013) article makes a particularly significant contribution towards pointing contemporary CP towards a clearer professional identity.

Conclusion

The professional practice of psychology in SA has been deeply influenced by the country's history of racial exclusion and economic exploitation. CP, by implication, has been complicit with the apartheid project. It was only in the 1980s that critical voices began to emerge calling attention to the racist and exclusionary character of the discipline which has resulted in some transformation. However, more than twenty years since SA became a democratic state, CPs are still predominantly White and still serve a mainly elite clientele. The specialty thus faces a number of challenges, which include finding ways to provide psychological interventions which are accessible, relevant, far-reaching and evidenced based. This will require a shift from one-on-one interventions to broad-based community and public health interventions – an area where CP in SA can make a significant contribution, providing that a suitable funding model can be found and posts are created within the public health care system. In this context we note developments with the National Health Insurance scheme spearheaded by the current Minister of Health which will no doubt have an impact on the practice of CP in SA. Our position on blurring the distinction between clinical and CP warrants ongoing discussion and debate. We maintain that contestations about turf and scope of practice are unnecessary and unproductive as they perpetuate divisions in the field and prohibit services from being rendered effectively while drawing attention away from much more serious issues such as the mental health treatment gap in SA and the need for evidence-based practices.

Disclosure statement

No potential conflict of interest was reported by the authors.

References

Abrahams, N., Jewkes, R., Martin, L. J., Mathews, S., Vetten, L., & Lombard, C. (2009). Mortality of women from intimate partner violence in South Africa: A national epidemiological study. *Violence and Victims, 24*, 546–556.

American Psychological Association. (2015). *Policy statement on evidence-based practice in psychology.* Retrieved from http://www.apa.org/practice/guidelines/evidence-based-statement.aspx

Ammassari, A., Trotta, M. P., Murri, R., Castelli, F., Narciso, P., Noto, P., … Antinori, A. (2002). Correlates and predictors of adherence to highly active antiretroviral therapy: Overview of published literature. *JAIDS Journal of Acquired Immune Deficiency Syndromes, 31*, S123–S127.

Bedi, R. P., Haverkamp, B. E., Beatch, R., Cave, D. G., Domene, J. F., Harris, G. E., & Mikhail, A. M. (2011). Counselling psychology in a Canadian context: Definition and description. *Canadian Psychology/Psychologie canadienne, 52*, 128–138.

Bolton, P., Bass, J., Betancourt, T., Speelman, L., Onyango, G., Clougherty, K. F., … Verdeli, H. (2007). Interventions for depression symptoms among adolescent survivors of war and displacement in Northern Uganda. *Journal of the American Medical Association, 298*, 519–527.

Bolton, P., Bass, J., Neugebauer, R., Verdeli, H., Clougherty, K. F., Wickramaratne, P., … Weissman, M. (2003). Group interpersonal psychotherapy for depression in rural Uganda. *Journal of the American Medical Association, 289*, 3117–3124.

Botha, E. (2011, June 13). Psychologists on war path. *Times Live*. Retrieved May 3, 2013, from http://www.timeslive.co.za/lifestyle/health/2011/06/13/psychologists-on-war-path

Catz, S. L., Kelly, J. A., Bogart, L. M., Benotsch, E. G., & McAuliffe, T. L. (2000). Patterns, correlates, and barriers to medication adherence among persons prescribed new treatments for HIV disease. *Health Psychology, 19*, 124.

Cook, J., & Visser, B. (1986). Counseling psychology. *Kompas/Compass, 9*, 1–2.

Cooper, S. (2014). A synopsis of South African psychology from apartheid to democracy. *American Psychologist, 69*, 837–847.

Cooper, S., Nicholas, L., Seedat, M., & Statman, J. (1990). Psychology and apartheid: The struggle for psychology in South Africa. In L. J. Nicholas & S. Cooper (Eds.), *Psychology and apartheid: Essays on the struggle and the mind in South Africa* (pp. 1–21). Johannesburg: Vision/Madiba Press.

de la Rey, C., & Ipser, J. (2004). The call for relevance: South African psychology ten years into democracy. *South African Journal of Psychology, 34*, 544–552.

Department of Health. (2012). *Annual report 2012/2013 (No. 237/2012)*. Retrieved from http://africacheck.org/wp-content/uploads/2014/02/131016dohrreport.pdf

Foster, D. (1993). On racism: Virulent mythologies and fragile threads. In L. J. Nicholas (Ed.), *Psychology and oppression: Critiques and proposals* (pp. 55–80). Johannesburg: Skotaville.

Foster, D. (2004). Liberation psychology. In N. Duncan (Ed.), *Self, community and psychology* (pp. 1.1–1.44). Cape Town: UCT Press.

Freeman, M., Nkomo, N., Kafaar, Z., & Kelly, K. (2008). Mental disorder in people living with HIV/AIDS in South Africa. *South African Journal of Psychology, 38*, 489–500.

Freeman, M., Patel, V., Collins, P. Y., & Bertolote, J. (2005). Integrating mental health in global initiatives for HIV/AIDS. *The British Journal of Psychiatry, 187*(1), 1–3.

Goodyear, R. K., Lichtenberg, J. W., Hutman, H., Overland, E., Bedi, R., Christiani, K., ... Young, C. (in press). A global portrait of counselling psychologists' characteristics, perspectives, and professional behaviors. *Counselling Psychology Quarterly*. doi: 10.1080/09515070.2015.1128396

Goodyear, R. K., Murdock, N., Lichtenberg, J. W., McPherson, R., Koetting, K., & Petren, S. (2008). Stability and change in counseling psychologists' identities, roles, functions, and career satisfaction across 15 years. *The Counseling Psychologist, 36*, 220–249.

Government Gazette. (1974). *Law on doctors, dentists and supplementary health professions, No. 56 of 1974*. Pretoria: Government Printer.

Government Gazette. (2011). *Regulations defining the scope of the profession of psychology (No. 34581)*. Retrieved from http://www.hpcsa.co.za/Uploads/editor/UserFiles/downloads/psych/sept_promulgated_scope_of_practice.pdf

Health Professions Act 56. (1974). Retrieved from http://www.hpcsa.co.za/Uploads/editor/UserFiles/downloads/legislations/acts/health_professions_ct_56_1974.pdf

Herman, A. A., Stein, D. J., Seedat, S., Heeringa, S. G., Moomal, H., & Williams, D. R. (2009). The South African stress and health (SASH) study: 12-month and lifetime prevalence of common mental disorders. *South African Medical Journal, 99*, 339–344.

HPCSA. (2013a). *Education and training*. Retrieved from http://www.hpcsa.co.za/PBPsychology/Education

HPCSA. (2013b). *iRegister*. Retrieved from http://isystems.hpcsa.co.za/iregister/

Igreja, V., Kleijn, W. C., Schreuder, B. J. N., van Dijk, J. A., & Verschuur, M. (2004). Testimony method to ameliorate post-traumatic stress symptoms. Community-based intervention study with Mozambican civil war survivors. *The British Journal of Psychiatry, 184*, 251–257.

Kagee, A. (2006). Where is the evidence in South African clinical psychology? *South African Journal of Psychology, 36*, 233–248.

Kalichman, S., Simbayi, L., Jooste, S., Toefy, Y., Cain, D., Cherry, C., & Kagee, A. (2005). Development of a brief scale to measure AIDS-related stigma in South Africa. *AIDS and Behavior, 9*, 135–143.

Kaminer, D., Grimsrud, A., Myer, L., Stein, D. J., & Williams, D. R. (2008). Risk for post-traumatic stress disorder associated with different forms of interpersonal violence in South Africa. *Social Science & Medicine, 67*, 1589–1595.

Leach, M. M., Akhurst, J., & Basson, C. (2003). Counseling psychology in South Africa: Current political and professional challenges and future promise. *The Counseling Psychologist, 31*, 619–640.

Minaar, A., Pretorius, S., & Wentzel, M. (1995). Who goes there? Illegals in South Africa. *Indicator SA, 12*, 33–40.

Neuner, F., Onyut, P. L., Ertl, V., Odenwald, M., Schauer, E., & Elbert, T. (2008). Treatment of posttraumatic stress disorder by trained lay counselors in an African refugee settlement: A randomized controlled trial. *Journal of Consulting and Clinical Psychology, 76*, 686–694.

Olley, B. O., Seedat, S., Nei, D. G., & Stein, D. J. (2004). Predictors of major depression in recently diagnosed patients with HIV/AIDS in South Africa. *AIDS Patient Care and STDs, 18*, 481–487.

Packard, T. (2009). The 2008 Leona Tyler award address: Core values that distinguish counseling psychology: Personal and professional perspectives. *The Counseling Psychologist, 37*, 610–624.

Painter, D., & Terre Blanche, M. (2004). Critical psychology in South Africa: Looking back and looking ahead. *South African Journal of Psychology: South African Psychology: Reviewing the First Decade of Democracy: Special Issue, 34*, 520–543.

Pelling, N. (2004). Counselling psychology: Diversity and commonalities across the western world. *Counselling Psychology Quarterly, 17*, 239–245.

Pillay, Y. G., & Petersen, I. (1996). Current practice patterns of clinical and counselling psychologists and their attitudes to transforming mental health polices in South Africa. *South African Journal of Psychology, 26*, 76–80.

Savickas, M. L. (2007). *Reshaping the story of career counselling. Shaping the story – A guide to facilitating narrative counselling* (pp. 1–3). Pretoria: Van Schaik.

Seedat, S., Williams, D. R., Herman, A. A., Moomal, H., Williams, S. L., Jackson, P. B., ... Stein, D. J. (2009). Mental health service use among South Africans for mood, anxiety and substance use disorders. *South African Medical Journal , 99*, 346–352.

Seekings, J., & Nattrass, N. (2006). *Class, race and inequality in South Africa.* Pietermaritzburg: UKZN Press.

Spire, B., Duran, S., Souville, M., Leport, C., Raffi, F., & Moatti, J. P. (2002). Adherence to highly active antiretroviral therapies (HAART) in HIV-infected patients: From a predictive to a dynamic approach. *Social Science & Medicine, 54*, 1481–1496.

Stead, G. B., & Watson, M. B. (2006). Indigenisation of psychology in South Africa. In G. B. Stead & M. B. Watson (Eds.), *Career psychology in the South African context* (pp. 214–225). Pretoria: Van Schaik.

The World Bank. (2015). *Population, total.* Retrieved from http://data.worldbank.org/indicator/SP.POP.TOTL

Turner, B. J., Laine, C., Cosler, L., & Hauck, W. W. (2003). Relationship of gender, depression, and health care delivery with antiretroviral adherence in HIV-infected drug users. *Journal of General Internal Medicine, 18*, 248–257.

UNHCR. (1951). Convention and protocol relating to the status of refugees. Retrieved from http://www.unhcr.org/3b66c2aa10.html

Van Ommen, C., & Painter, D. (Eds.). (2008). *Interiors: A history of psychology in South Africa.* Pretoria: Unisa Press.

Vera, E. M., & Speight, S. L. (2003). Multicultural competence, social justice, and counseling psychology: Expanding our roles. *The Counseling Psychologist, 31*, 253–272.

Watson, M. B., & Fouche, P. (2007). Transforming a past into a future: Counseling psychology in South Africa. *Applied Psychology, 56*, 152–164.

Young, C. (2013). South African counselling psychology at the crossroads: Lessons to be learned from around the world. *South African Journal of Psychology, 43*, 422–433.

Young, I. M. (1990). *Justice and the politics of difference*. Princeton, NJ: Princeton University Press.

Counselling psychology in South Korea

Young A. Ju[a], Young-joo Han[a], Hyejin Lee[b] and Dong-gwi Lee[c]

[a]Korea Counseling Graduate University, Seoul, South Korea; [b]NdyneINC Corp., Seoul, South Korea; [c]Department of Psychology, Yonsei University, Seoul, South Korea

Counselling psychology (CP) in South Korea has grown tremendously as it establishes its unique niche in the mental health profession. Diverse practice under the roof of CP is a strength as well as a weakness. In this paper, we describe the characteristics of CP in South Korea in terms of history, credentialing, the service delivery system, organizations, training, distinctive features from other adjacent areas, core values, and the profession's unique challenges and future directions. Future tasks include the establishment of clear professional identity, achievement of a governmental licensure system, a nationwide accreditation system, development of Korean-specific ways of counselling, protocols for trauma, and increased accessibility.

Counselling psychology (CP) in South Korea has over 60 years' history, beginning with the influx of Western counselling and psychotherapy in the early 1950s. A dramatic expansion in the number of counsellors has taken place; in the period of 1987–2015, the number of counselling psychologists has increased drastically from 20 to over 20,000. The terms "counselling psychologists" and "counsellors" are used interchangeably throughout this paper since the distinction between the two in South Korea is not often made. We discuss across eight key aspects of CP: (a) its history, (b) current credential systems, (c) its place in the health delivery system, (d) professional organizations, (e) training programmes, (f) its relationship to other adjacent health care providers, (g) traditions and core values and (h) major issues facing the profession.

A brief history of CP in South Korea

The Korean counselling profession finds its roots in the work of the American Education Mission (AEM) which provided educational aids to rebuild the Korean War-damaged education system. AEM's primary work included teacher education and educational curriculum development. Following the AEM's recommendations, the Korean Central Education Research Institute developed the area of student guidance and counselling. In line with this, in 1957 Seoul's Board of Education provided training courses for adjustment guidance teachers. The term "guidance" was used and basic counselling activities were incorporated into the coursework.

In 1962, Ewha Woman's University Guidance Center was founded, the first counselling institute for college students. The next year, the Korean Counselor Association[1] was formed, the first association for professional counsellors. In 1973, the Department of Correction issued the "Regulations for Education Act," which provided a legal basis for counselling activities. In addition, Seoul's Board of Education instituted a programme from 1985 to 1988 to routinely train and allocate counsellors to secondary schools. The initiative – with a strong focus on counselling for students and adolescents – provided a basis for the formation of "the Square for Youths' Conversation" under the Korean government in 1993 (renamed the Korea Youth Counseling Institute in 1999 and then the Korea Youth Counseling and Welfare Institute in 2012).

By 1975, two major universities in Seoul (Ewha Woman's University in 1972 and Seoul National University in 1975) offered CP as an independent, graduate major. Before that, CP was provided as part of the curriculum for a general liberal arts major. Another important component in the history of South Korean CP can be found in its strong emphasis on group counselling. Cheon, Seul, and Bae (2004) reported that Ho Kyun Yun conducted the first group counselling (a T-group) in South Korea in 1970 at the Central Institute of Student Guidance. A year later, Sang Hoon Lee, a teacher who offered sensitivity training in school settings, formed a special interest group on group counselling. In 1989 it developed into the Korea Institute of Counseling. Hyung-Deuk Lee also organized T-groups for various clienteles including graduate students, housewives and Protestant clergymen. These initial efforts formed the foundations of such group counselling associations as the Korea Institute of Developmental Counseling (1990), the Korean Group Counseling Association (1998) and the Han Counseling Association (launched by Dong-Su Yoo in 2003). Group counselling with a focus on sensitivity training has been one of South Korean CP's unique efforts both to serve the public and to foster counsellor trainees' awareness.

Tao Psychotherapy is another force that influenced the growth of South Korean CP. Dongshick Rhee, a psychiatrist, proposed it in the mid-1970s specifically for Koreans as an integration of Eastern Tao (Taoism, Buddhism and Confucianism), indigenous Korean culture and Western psychotherapy. Its main focus is to help clients to be aware of their nuclear emotions and to relieve their discomfort (Rhee, 1990). In 1979, the Korean Academy of Psychotherapists (KAP) was founded to facilitate the refinement of Tao Psychotherapy, with many counselling psychologist as members (e.g. Jahng-Ho Lee, Ho Kyun Yun, and Hae-Rim Choi).

Finally and importantly, the Division of Counseling and Psychotherapy (DCP) separated from the Korean Psychological Association's Division of Clinical Psychology in 1987. The separation was fuelled by counsellors' strong desire to conduct psychotherapy rather than to be limited to assessment and psychological testing in hospital settings. The counsellors who founded the DCP worked to explore effective psychotherapy techniques through monthly case conferences. The DCP changed its name to the Korean Counseling and Psychotherapy Association in 1996 and then became the Korean Counseling Psychological Association (KCPA) in 2003 and has remained so since. Some KCPA members founded the Korean Counseling Association (KCA), with narrower focus on education, in 2000. South Korean CP now is supported mainly by these two associations through their collaboration and competition. In 2013 KCPA and KCA formed a consortium (the Mental Health Counselor Council) with two other groups, the Korean Association of Family Therapy (KAFT), and Korean Association of Christian Counseling and Psychotherapy (KACCP) to work together towards government licensure of CPs.

Credentialing and registration

Whereas the Ministry of Mental Health and Welfare licenses clinical psychologists and social workers, South Korea has no official governmental licence for CPs who work across all age groups. The only government-issued licence available for CPs is that of "Youth Counsellors," who are certified by the Korean Youth Counseling and Welfare Institute (KYCWI).

KCPA, KCA, KAFT and KACCP all offer counsellor certificate systems. For example, KCPA issues the certificates for both "Level-1 Counselor" (at least 5 years' training) and "Level-2 Counselor" (3 years' training). Similarly, the KCA has four levels of counsellor certificates (Professional Counselor Level-1, 2 and 3 and Supervisor-level Counselor). Both associations provide qualifying examinations, training and continuing education for certified counsellors.

Public counselling service delivery system

The counselling service delivery system in South Korea is organized by the government. The Korean government provides public services through three levels. The government agencies (Level 1) either provide services themselves or manage the services offered at Level 2 (organizations founded by legislations) and Level 3 (educational institutes including counselling centres). In specific, Level 1 agencies involve the Ministry of Gender Equality and Family (MGEF); Ministry of Education, Science and Technology (MEST); Ministry of National Defense (MND); Ministry of Employment and Labor (MEL); and Ministry of Health and Welfare (MHW). These departments plan and develop policies regarding the overall structures and flows of the counselling services. Level 2 includes the Korea Youth Counseling and Welfare Institute and Center for Employment and Labor. These organizations either operate counselling businesses in practice or support counselling centres on the front line.

The aforementioned five governmental agencies make available various counselling services with different business targets and methods. First, the MGEF handles counselling services in particular for youths outside of school, families and women. For example, the MGEF implements policies to assist at-risk youth through the KYCWI, which has founded Youth Counseling and Welfare Centers. These centres have served as a hub to provide services for youth at risk within their local communities. In addition, these centres have established more localized service providers, such as "My Dream Centers (MDC)" that provides youths with services including personal counselling, psycho-education, career exploration, assistance with job search and recruitment and self-sufficiency support.

Second, the MEST generally governs policies related to students' welfare within the school. "Wee Centers", units of Office of Education Support in cities, are the most representative example of their work. Wee Centers, under the Law for Prevention and

Countermeasure of School Violence, focus on the prevention of school violence and counselling services for students at risk with severe mental illness.

Third, the MND governs military counselling. This service is managed by the "Korean Defense Investigative Agency (KDIA)" at the second level and provided by Military Camp Counsellors at the lowest level, specializing in assisting soldiers with adjustment and promoting their welfare. Also, under the budget of the KDIA, "National Defense Help Call 1303" through the "Military Police ARS System", provides phone counselling for soldiers and military personnel having difficulties with their military services.

Fourth, the MEL has subordinate units such as the Bureau of a Manpower Supply and Demand which make plans for effective employment and job-seeking activities. The Centers for Employment and Labor in each regional unit provide job-related counselling, vocational training and job placement services.

Finally, the MHW tasks the Bureau of Health Policy with mental health. Front-line services are offered by Mental Health Promotion Centers in affiliation with local governments as well as university hospitals. Counselling-related services provided by these centres mostly involve treatments with medications. Usually clinical psychologists, rather than counselling psychologists, work at these centres to perform psychological testing and diagnosis.

The major professional CP organizations

KCPA has the longest history, the largest number of members and the most public credibility of the four Korean counselling associations. Since its inauguration in 1964 as the second Division of the Korean Psychological Association (KPA), KCPA has grown to have the largest membership of any of KPA's 15 original Divisions. As of 2015, the number of individual members with a master's or higher degrees in a counselling-related major exceeds 20,000. More than 1000 KCPA members hold its Level-1 Counsellor certificate; over 3500 hold its Level-2 Counsellor certificate. The KCPA website states the responsibility of its members as: "Each and every KCPA member strives to learn and develop theories and practice of counselling and psychotherapy to improve mental health of the society and to prevent and treat problems that an individual suffers from in a rapidly-changing society". Also, the KCPA has 11 standing committees and publishes the *Korean Journal of Psychology: Counseling and psychotherapy.*

Training programmes and accreditation systems

Counsellor training programmes in South Korea are operated autonomously by each university and organization, and therefore lack a unified system (Choi & Kim, 2006; Song, Kim, Kim, & Lee, 2012). However, KCPA has "institution members" that are authorized through its certification system to run counsellor training programmes as well as official case conferences. KCA provides an even more robust and widespread system to screen and authorize counsellor training programmes and institutions. By November 2014, KCA had approved 188 institutions, as compared to the 69 KCPA had approved as of August 2015. The training institutions KCA authorizes are required to go through a mandatory reaccreditation procedure every 5 years. KCA training programmes include an internship programme, training programmes for personal counselling, professional training programmes for group counselling, special lectures and workshops on psychological tests, parental education and education for sex counsellors and youth counsellors.

Traditions, core values and the identity of CP in South Korea

South Korean CP is in a transitional status where it is establishing its professional identity in the context of Korean culture. Although CP in South Korea adopted Western psychotherapy theories, those have limitations when applied to Korean culture. In response, Korean CPs have developed counselling theories that incorporate traditional Korean philosophy (e.g. "Han" counselling and Tao psychotherapy) and are continuing to discuss culturally sensitive counselling practices.

Studies (e.g. Kim, Kwon, Han, & Sohn, 2008; Lee, Yang, & Seo, 2007) suggest that Korean counselling, in contrast to Western counselling, is more directive and educational. Moreover, the counselling relationship in Korea is more hierarchical and collectivistic with an emphasis on "we" rather than "I" (Chang, 2002; Kim et al., 2008) than is true in the West. This may stem from the influence of Confucianism where "Hyo" (children's respect and care for their parents) and "Chung" (people's loyalty to their king and country) are emphasized. Given that, in Korean counselling, clients often expect counsellors to provide them with not only emotional support, but also direction and guidance which they might otherwise receive from their parents. Relatedly, then, Chang (2002) argued that when counsellors assist clients with restoring the parent–children relationship, the effects of counselling can be enhanced.

In Korean society, however, both conservative generations who are influenced by traditional Confucianism and progressive generations who received modern democratic educations coexist. Thus, a unilateral application of traditional Korean values into counselling is inadequate. For instance, Han and O'Brien (2014) found that Korean clients may initially expect an authoritative counsellor whom they can admire as a respectable senior. But as the therapeutic relationship progresses, the effect of counselling can be enhanced when the counsellor–client relationship becomes an equal partnership.

An imminent task for Korean counselling is to help Korean society – where uniformity as an ethnically homogenous nation is typically assumed – to embrace and adjust to increasing diversity. Another challenge is addressing clients' unrealistic expectations that may hinder effectiveness. For instance, some clients expect their problems to be resolved through one or two counselling sessions with a diagnosis-and-prescription process. Others avoid help seeking as they see counselling centres as a place for those with psychological problems and therefore stigmatizing. An important task for South Korean CP is to educate people to develop appropriate expectations and perceptions for counselling (Yoo, 2005).

Comparison between counselling psychology and related professions

Differences between CP and other adjacent professions (clinical psychology and social work) in South Korea can be best described by their respective clienteles, work roles and work/training sites. CPs work primarily with members of the general population who seek psychological help to solve an array of life problems in relation to personality, aptitude, intelligence and career (as well as physical, emotional and behavioural symptoms; Lee & Lee, 2014). The work roles of counselling psychologists include providing: (a) remedial interventions to help clients to identify and resolve their problems towards growth; (b) psycho-educations to reduce the adverse effects from traumatic experiences; and (c) prevention programmes for people at risk (e.g. juvenile delinquents, youth self-injury and couples in crisis). CPs are found in counselling centres, private companies, schools and local communities.

On the other hand, clinical psychologists serve patients suffering from more severe mental problems. They offer assessment and diagnosis for mental illness by utilizing psychological tests, as well as provide clinical treatments for people in serious emotional distress (Ahn, 2010). Clinical psychologists usually work at mental hospitals and mental health centres.

Lastly, social workers are the professionals who plan, implement and evaluate various social welfare programmes necessary for general and clinical populations. Once social workers identify individuals or communities who are in need of assistance, they provide them not only with material support as needed but also educational guidance to better their current situations. To put together diverse resources and establish a more integrated support system, social workers work with various people and organizations such as researchers and personnel at national research institutions, welfare foundations, corporate social responsibility teams, social welfare institutions and health and medical institutions (Kim, 2004).

In short, CPs are more likely than clinical psychologists to work with clients vs. patients, in schools and counselling centres vs. hospitals and to employ growth-oriented vs. remedial models. And whereas CPs aim to help individual clients and a small group of people through psychotherapy, social workers conduct case studies to locate individuals in need of support and provide necessary resources in collaboration with various supporters.

Given that the expanding number of people in crisis and who present with progressively more complicated life problems, collaboration among the three professions is increasingly demanded. However, such professional collaboration is challenging for CPs as they have not yet obtained a stable, legal status as professional mental health service providers. Although the current laws in South Korea often use "psychological counselling" to describe general counselling services, they do not specify counselling psychologists as persons who can provide those services but laws instead specify clinical psychologists and social workers.

For example, under article 17 of the Children's Welfare Law: counsellors for Child Protection Institutions, counsellors must hold one of the following: (a) having a certification of "Level-1 Social Worker"; (b) having a university degree in psychology (including welfare psychology) or equivalent or higher from a school, or (c) completion of academic courses related to children's welfare or social welfare. Article 17 does not recognize CPs as legitimately qualified professionals in this area. On the other hand, the Children's Welfare Law provides a standard regarding the qualifications for the professionals who can conduct psychological treatments including "counselling" who are described as "clinical psychotherapy professionals.

Major issues, opportunities and concerns for CP in South Korea

Although the demands for counselling have brought a dramatic increase in the number of counsellor trainees, significant challenges still exist. The most important are: (a) further refinement of the identity of CP and role of counselling psychologists; (b) establishment of a governmental licensure and accreditation system; (c) continuing education for counsellors while preventing burnout; and (d) expanding accessibility to counselling services for the public.

Further refinement of the identity of CP and role of counselling psychologists

A challenge remains concerning the difficulty of defining the identity and role of South Korean CP. This is particularly true for counselling psychologists when compared with other adjacent mental health professionals such as clinical psychologists, social workers, psychotherapists and art therapists. At the extreme end of professionalism, fortunetellers in South Korea may present themselves as life counsellors. The Korean word meaning "counselling" is a generic term that describes any behaviours to offer counsel to people who seek information or help (e.g. financial solution, information about military, etc.), and thus, many professionals with various expertise would prefer to be called "a counsellor".

Further, the pioneers who separated the Counseling and Psychotherapy Division (CPD) from that of Clinical Psychology made efforts to embrace mental health professionals from various backgrounds under the umbrella of CP by having different requirements for status as a counselling psychologist. This approach had pros and cons. The bright side takes pride in the dramatic increase in the number of counselling psychologists or counsellors. As mentioned earlier, in 1987 the CPD founding members numbered only 20, while in 2015 the membership office of the same division counts over 17,000 counsellors. On the other hand, Gelso and Fretz (1992) raise, "the identity problem of counseling psychology ... (are any of us absolutely sure of who we are?)" (p. 41). It is not straightforward to define what South Korean CP is or what counselling psychologists do. Different counselling associations provide different definitions of counselling, roles as a counsellor, core values and training models. Such heterogeneity confuses not only the Korean government which needs to screen and hire professional counsellors, but also people who are in need of quality counselling services. Back in 1999, Naomi Meara advocated the term, "unified diversity," defined as "embracing diversity and finding strength in it" (Gelso & Fretz, 1992, p. 43) to argue that diversity in CP is not a weakness but rather a unique strength if the profession itself values and embraces it. Given that, one crucial question that lies in South Korean CP is whether the profession can achieve "unified diversity" while maintaining the core values and unique expertise of CP. Furthermore, as Park and Hwang (2008) cogently suggest, unique values and training models are required to resolve the identity issue. As mentioned earlier, some examples that have been discussed in this context include (a) "Tao-Psychotherapy" (Dongshick Rhee, 1990), (b) "Onmeum[2] Counseling" (Yun, 2007) that highlights the importance of differentiating clients' imagination from their reality itself through concentrated meditation based on Buddhism and (c) "Reality Dynamic Counseling" (Chang, 2002) that advocates a unique Korean counsellor role of "a strict father and loving mother" who can guide clients with realistic perspectives based on a parent–child relationship in Korea. More work is needed to establish an integrated model of South Korean CP with its values of eastern beliefs, collectivism and strong relationship orientation.

Establishment of governmental licensure and accreditation

As described above, a clear challenge for South Korean counselling profession resides in its lack of governmental approval of counsellor certificates issued by the KCPA and KCA. This is a complicated issue since the MHW in South Korea has refused the approval of the mental health counsellor licence for CP practitioners. The rationale for disapproval is twofold; first, that the MHW already has approved several mental health-related licences (such as mental health clinical psychologist and mental health social worker), and thus they fail to find a good reason to add another licence for counsellors; and second, since the bulk of counselling associations issue counselling certificates on their own, it is hard to screen a qualified certificate from an unqualified one. Relatedly, frequent competition for hegemony among the counselling associations often has made the MHW unwilling to take sides. Fortunately, four counselling associations (KCPA, KCP, KAFT and KACCP) formed a consortium ("Mental Health Counselor Council") that has the promise to address this.

Another challenge for the South Korean counselling profession involves its lack of a unified accreditation system for counsellor training programmes. This is a critical limitation, since the quality of training can fluctuate with the level of competence each training site possesses. Because of great heterogeneity in training sites and systems, it is hard to set up a common guideline for successful and sufficient training. In this realm, Choi and Kim (2006) suggested: (a) development of a quality graduate curriculum for counsellor trainees with a focus on enhancing clinical competence, (b) establishment of a consortium among graduate programmes to share training resources and (c) an increase in collaboration between graduate programmes and counselling associations to provide continuing education for counsellors.

Continuing education for counsellors while preventing burnout

It is important to find ways to encourage more widespread and systematic use of continuing education. On the one hand, it is understandable that counsellors may feel resistance to fulfil another burden after all their hard work to receive certification. But without continuing education, it is not possible for them to keep up with advancements in counselling. The KCA has developed a system for continuing education to maintain and develop counsellors' competency. Since the Korean suicide rate now ranks first among the OECD countries, the roles of counsellors have come to the forefront. With this national trust in their hands, it is not an option but a necessity to provide quality continuing education for Korean counsellors.

As society grows complicated, clients bring more complex problems to the counselling context. Even master counsellors experience burnout including symptoms of physical fatigue, feelings of helplessness, lack of support at work, diminished interest in clients and blurred boundaries between personal and professional lives (see Lee et al., 2008). Counsellors who frequently work with adolescents, often called "Youth Companions" in South Korea, report their agony and burnout symptoms (Choi, Son, & Lee, 2013). Continuing education has an important role to play in helping counsellors to prevent and cope with possible burnout, to enable them to continue to contribute to the welfare of their clients as well as society.

An area that necessitates continuing education for South Korean counsellors is crisis intervention. Recent disasters such as the sinking of MV Sewol (the morning of 16 April 2014) and the MERS breakout presented South Korean counsellors with new challenges, as most have not been trained specifically for crisis counselling or trauma resolution. Needed is an effort to advance Korean counsellors' competence across several areas, such as an understanding of trauma victims (Cheon, 2014), crisis intervention (e.g. Lee, 2005), trauma resolution therapy (e.g. Greenwald, 2002) and models of collaboration with other professionals. Earlier in 2015, the KCA has launched the "Support Counsellor Group for People in Disaster" to address this issue.

Expanding accessibility to counselling services

One challenge is to help clients in need to get access to counselling services. Currently, several hurdles impede clients from accessing services. Most importantly, it is not convenient to locate the lists and names of qualified counsellors in South Korea. Their contact numbers are neither easily found in the phone book nor in advertisements. Because of that, many potential clients need to find an informant around them who can lead them to either counselling centres or specific counsellors they know of. More efforts are clearly needed in this area.

There is also a tendency that qualified counsellors are likely to spend more of their time supervising counsellor trainees than meeting with clients. By contrast, relatively beginner-level counsellors typically serve clients. This might be due to the great number of counsellor trainees who seek supervision, but clearly it is not a desirable situation for the greater body of clients who suffer from severe mental issues. This is almost certainly an outgrowth of the rapid expansion of the profession and is not easy to address.

An additional challenge for clients is the financial burden. Unlike other countries such as the United States where clients can get support from their insurance companies or help through a sliding scale, counselling fees are not covered by current medical insurance in Korea. This warrants developing ways to alleviate clients' financial burden in the near future.

Key articles

Only a few references on South Korean CP are available in English. We recommend the following references.

Lee, S. M., Suh, S., Yang, E., & Jang, Y. J. (2012). History, current status, and future prospects of counseling in South Korea. *Journal of Counseling & Development, 90*, 494–499.

Seo, Y. S., Kim, D. M., & Kim, D. I. (2007). Current status and prospects of Korean counseling psychology: Research, clinical training, and job placement. *Applied Psychology, 56*, 107–118.

Conclusion

CP in South Korea started with a strong emphasis on education and guidance in school settings. The work domains and clienteles of counselling psychologists have expanded to include families, women in crisis, military and youths at risk. And the focus of their work has evolved from a traditional, remedial intervention to both prevention and promotion of people's strengths and potentials. Over 60 years of history, South Korean CP has contributed to enhancing Koreans' mental health and welfare through various initiatives, which include intensive psychotherapy, group counselling, implementation of interventions and psycho-education, and advocacy for people in crisis. Continual efforts have also been made to develop Korean-specific ways of counselling. An imminent task for the profession is to persuade the Ministry of Mental Health and Welfare to include counselling psychologists as government-approved professionals who can work at mental health centres. The recent coordinated efforts of the "Mental Health Counselor Council" work towards this goal. It is desirable to establish an accreditation system for both undergraduate and graduate training programmes of counselling, which can help the profession to enhance its expertise and quality services. It is a hope that diversity among mental health professions is not a hurdle or a source of conflict but an asset which enriches the field. Of utmost importance for the profession is to best serve the Korean community. CP in South Korea is a distinctive helping profession.

Disclosure statement

No potential conflict of interest was reported by the authors.

Notes

1. Note the "Korean Counselor Association" differs from the "Korean Counseling Association" (KCA). The latter will be introduced later in this paper.
2. The meaning of this Korean word is "whole mindfulness."

References

Ahn, C.-Y. (2010). *Clinical psychology* (3rd ed.). Seoul: Sigmapress.

Chang, S.-S. (2002). The counselor character desired in Korean culture. *The Korean Journal of Counseling and Psychotherapy, 14*, 547–561.

Cheon, J.-K. (2014, June). An existential exploration of trauma victim's Life. *Korean Psychological Association: Annual Conference Program and Abstract, 1*, 163.

Cheon, S.-M., Seul, C.-D., & Bae, J.-W. (2004). The present status and task of group counseling in Korea. *Student Counseling Research, 5*, 61–74.

Choi, H.-R., & Kim, Y.-H. (2006). Study on the graduate curriculum for the counselor education and training programs in Korea. *The Korean Journal of Counseling and Psychotherapy, 18*, 713–729.

Choi, H.-A., Son, J.-Y., & Lee, E.-J. (2013). Relationships among job demand, burnout and turnover intentions of youth companion: The mediating effect of burnout. *Korean Journal of Counseling, 14*(1), 191–207.

Gelso, C. J., & Fretz, B. R. (1992). *Counseling psychology.* New York, NY: Harcourt Brace Jovanovich.

Greenwald, R. (2002). Motivation-adaptive skills-trauma resolution (MASTR) therapy for adolescents with conduct problems: An open trial. *Journal of Aggression, Maltreatment & Trauma, 6*, 237–261.

Han, Y. J., & O'Brien, K. M. (2014). Critical secret disclosure of psychotherapy with Korean clients. *The Counseling Psychologist, 42*, 1–29.

Kim, S.-K. (Ed.). (2004). *Introduction to social welfare.* Seoul: Nanam.

Kim, C.-D., Kwon, K.-I., Han, Y.-J., & Sohn, N.-H. (2008). The Korean counselor's factors which contribute to positive counseling outcomes. *Korean Journal of Counseling, 9*, 961–985.

Lee, Y.-J. (2005). Psychological studies of crisis from disaster. *Journal of Safety and Crisis Management, 1*, 85–99.

Lee, J.-H., & Lee, D.-G. (2014). *Counseling psychology* (5th ed.). Seoul: Parkyoung Story.

Lee, J., Nam, S., Park, H.-R., Kim, D.-H., Lee, M.-K., & Lee, S. M. (2008). The relationship between years of counseling experience and counselors' burnout: A comparative study of Korean and American counselors. *The Korean Journal of Counseling and Psychotherapy, 20*, 23–42.

Lee, E.-K., Yang, N.-M., & Seo, E.-K. (2007). A qualitative study on counseling in Korea. *The Korean Journal of Counseling and Psychotherapy, 19*, 587–607.

Park, A.-S., & Hwang, M.-G. (2008). Issues for identification in relation to counseling in Korea. *The Korean Journal of Counseling and Psychotherapy, 20*, 903–929.

Rhee, D. (1990). The tao, psychoanalysis and existential thought. *Psychotherapy and Psychosomatics, 53*, 21–27.

Song, J.-H., Kim, K.-S., Kim, B.-H., & Lee, H.-K. (2012). KCA members' needs for the improvement of qualification system for counseling specialist. *Korean Journal of Counseling, 13*, 1715–1729.

Yoo, S. K. (2005). Korean college students' attitudes toward counseling psychotherapy, and psychiatric help. *The Korean Journal of Counseling and Psychotherapy, 17*, 612–632.

Yun, H. K. (2007). The onmeum counseling. *The Korean Journal of Counseling and Psychotherapy, 19*, 505–522.

Development and current status of counselling psychology in Taiwan

Su-Fen Tu[a] and Shuh-Ren Jin[b]

[a]Graduate School of Education, Chung Yuan Christian University, Taoyuan City, Taiwan;
[b]Faculty of Education, University of Macau, Avenida da Universidade, Taipa, China

This article details the three stages of counselling psychology's development in Taiwan, including pre-legislation, legislation and post-legislation. In pre-legislation stage, a brief historical review of the growth of counselling and guidance is introduced, which is the root of the contemporary counselling psychology. The process of the Psychology Act's legislation is described in legislation stage and the relationships between counselling teachers and clinical psychologist are also discussed. In the post-legislation stage, the licensure system, training programmes, main professional organizations, work settings, and the major opportunities and challenges for the counselling psychology field are presented. In addition, the article refers to data from a national survey of 124 counselling psychologists to provide a profile of the counselling psychologists in Taiwan.

The watershed legislation for Taiwan counselling psychology (CP) has been the 2001 Psychologists' Act. It is so significant that the development of Taiwan's CP can be divided into three stages: pre-legislation, legislation and post-legislation.

Pre-legislation stage

After the Chinese Civil War ended in 1950, thousands of overseas students who were offspring of Chinese immigrants to other countries came to Taiwan to pursue their education. In response, the Regulations Regarding Study and Counselling Assistance for Overseas Chinese Students in Taiwan was introduced in 1958, enabling schools to provide guidance and counselling services to these students. In December of that same year, Dr Jiang Jian-Bai, an educator and senior administrator of Bureau of Education, founded the Chinese Guidance Association (CGA) under the support of the government. Jiang chaired the CGA board for 10 years and was honoured as the "Father of Taiwan Guidance" to highlight his tremendous contributions to the profession (Yeh, 2013).

CGA played a crucial role in the history of CP's development. It's major contributions included initiating guidance work for overseas Chinese students, promoting counselling and guidance education in middle schools, building counselling education class' curriculum standards, establishing the school counselling and guidance system and promoting career guidance in Taiwan's social welfare system (retrieved from http://www.guidance.org.tw/).

During this early stage, the government and CGA cooperated excellently in promoting counselling and guidance in Taiwan. Suggested by CGA and legislated by government, hundreds of laws, regulations and executive orders related to counselling and guidance were enforced in the school system (Yeh, 2013). For example, counselling sectors (including a counselling room, counsellor's offices, psychological testing packages) and curriculum (taught by trained counselling teachers) have become mandatory educational services in schools since the 1968 Primary and Junior High School Act. This Act created a counselling position in school system that was relatively unique in the world: this was the Counselling Teacher (CT), whose primary responsibilities were to nurture students' mental health through a weekly counselling curriculum, to intervene students' adjustment problems via psychological appraisals, individual and group counselling, and related administration work.

This top-down approach in implementing counselling roles and services made counselling and guidance a fast-growing specialty. However, the credibility of the counselling profession and the value of counselling service were questioned by other school teachers, students and parents due to the confounding roles of being simultaneously discipline regulator and counsellor, the lack of mental health awareness in society and the immaturity of counselling services (Lin, 2000; Wang, Kwan, & Huang, 2011; Yeh, 2013). The CTs were misperceived with "teacher" identity since they were all trained by teachers' colleges or universities with four-year undergraduate Guidance and Counselling courses. Therefore, the needs for "in-depth individual and group counselling" that helping students deal with "intra-psychic" issues evidently were unmet by the profession.

During 1980s–1990s, some pioneers who received CP training in the US in APA accredited programmes brought CP concepts and training models into the school counselling and guidance training programmes in Taiwan. This new trend of training models related to theories and practices of Western counselling psychotherapy had quickly brought vitality and change to the school guidance-based training programmes (Yeh, 2013). Except for the influence of Western psychotherapy, due to the heavy workloads in administration and teaching (normally 15–20 hours per week for guidance classes), many CTs made appeals to have more time focused on providing direct counselling services and made calls to have registered school counsellors and to introduce school-based CPs into the education systems (Hsiao & Jin, 1996).

In the pre-legislation stage, "counselling and guidance" was considered an educational service and has not gained its status or recognition as CP. It was cultivated in the land of Education (not the land of Psychology like many other countries), but grew up by obtaining its nourishments from CP. For the graduates who served in school settings, they called themselves as a "Counselling Teacher", or as a "Counsellor" for those who practiced in other community settings.

Legislation stage

The legislation that provided legal legitimacy for counselling psychologists surprised many of them in terms of the speed with which it was enacted. The clinical psychology branch of the Chinese Psychology Association (CPA) formed a task force in 1995 to promote legislation for clinical psychologists, but gained little attention, let alone progress (Lin & Hsu, 2008). However, the urgent demand for qualified mental health professionals became a public concern when a series of traumatic events (earthquake, air crash, typhoon floods, etc.) and social problems happened in Taiwan in the late 1990s resulted in societal pressures (Wang et al., 2011). Seizing the opportunity, CPA invited CGA as a partner to incorporate Clinical Psychologists and CPs under one umbrella entitled the Psychologists' Act. In March 2000, the CGA council, led by Dr Jin Shuh-Ren, began building a consensus among scholars and professionals from training institutes and major professional groups regarding the importance and substance of leg-islation. On 15 April 2000, a task force comprising 11 representatives was formed as the CP division in CGA. This should be the official birth of the term "Counselling Psy-chology" in Taiwan. The CP division's initial mission was to study the licensure system with regard to educational training, internship, certification and practice of CP.

Although counselling and guidance professionals were trained according to the counselling discipline as advocated in US, they were not considered a specialty under the psychology roof in Taiwan. So, it was understandable that counselling professionals struggled to accept as a part of "the psychologists" family and to be included in the law during the initial stages of the legislation process. On 24 April 2001, Legislator Lai Ching-De gathered 14 representatives of CPA and CGA, who negotiated a statute that included both clinical and counselling psychology (Lin & Hsu, 2008). The two spe-cialties share similar scopes of practice (Table 1), but psychological assessment and psychotherapy for psychosis and cerebral mental functions were the practice area exclu-sively for clinical psychologists. The Psychologists' Act was passed by the legislature on 31 October 2001 and was promulgated on 21 November 2001. The Act regulates the examination, licencing, business scope, and general duties of licenced psychologist, and mandates licence management and penalties for violating the act. On 14 December 2001, the Ministry of Examination conducted the first session of the National Psycholo-gist Examination. This gave legal recognition of CP as a psychology profession and a promising specialty in Taiwan.

The separation of counselling psychologists from counselling teachers

The legislative recognition of counselling psychologists (CPs) brought some conflicts between CPs and CTs. First, the Act defined CPs as medical professionals, which some-what shifted the normal-developmental emphasis of counselling training into a more psychopathology-based training. The exclusion of CTs from the national examination resulted in them unrecognized and the loss of any identity as CPs (Wang et al., 2011). As a result, the CTs endeavoured to restore their identities and professions in school settings, establishing the Counselling Teachers Association and promoting the Student Guidance and Counselling Act.[1]

Identity formation of counselling psychologists

Traditionally, Taiwan's CPs focused on normal-developmental approach and worked in school and community settings, whereas clinical psychologists trained with psychopathology approach and worked jointly with psychiatrists in medical settings,

Table 1. The comparison between counselling psychologists and clinical psychologists.

Basis	Counselling psychologists	Clinical psychologists
Scope of practice (The Psychologists' Act, 2001)	(1) Psychological assessment of general mental state and functions (2) Psychological counselling and psychotherapy for deviation and disturbances in psychological development, social adaptation or cognition, emotions, behaviours, etc (3) Psychological counselling and psychotherapy for neurosis (4) Other elective items relating to counselling psychology	(1) Psychological assessment of general mental state and functions (2) Psychological counselling and psychotherapy for deviation and disturbances in psychological development, social adaptation or cognition, emotions, behaviours, etc (3) Psychological counselling and psychotherapy for neurosis (4) Psychological assessment and psychotherapy for psychosis[a] (5) Psychological assessment and psychotherapy for cerebral mental functions[a] (6) Other elective items relating to clinical psychology
Examination subjects (Exam Rules, amend 2013)	(1) The psychology foundation of counselling (2) Theories of counselling & psychotherapy (3) The practice of counselling & psychotherapy and professional ethics (4) Mental health and abnormal psychology (5) Case evaluation and psychological assessment (6) Group counselling & psychotherapy	(1) The foundation knowledge of clinical psychology (2) The clinical psychology-general I (including the definition, description, and ontology of deviation behaviours) (3) The clinical psychology-general II (including psychological assessment and psychotherapy) (4) The clinical psychology-specialized I (including assessment and psychotherapy related to suicidal, violent behaviour, substance abuse and personality and adjustment disorders) (5) The clinical psychology-specialized II (including assessment and psychotherapy related to intellectual, psychosis and developmental disorders) (6) The clinical psychology-specialized III (including assessment and psychotherapy related to eating disorders, neurosis and stress – related disorders)

(*Continued*)

Table 1.   (*Continued*).

Basis	Counselling psychologists	Clinical psychologists
Internship programmes (Enforcement rules, amend 2011)	(1) The internship activities include (a) individual, marriage or family counselling and psychotherapy; (b) group counselling and psychotherapy; (c) case evaluation and psychological assessment; (d) psychological counselling, mental health education and preventive promotion work; (e) professional administration for counselling psychology institutions or agencies; (f) other elective items relating to counselling psychology	(1) The internship items are the same as the scope of practice
	(2) The internship shall be conducted under the supervision of a counselling psychologist who has been practicing for two years, or more	(2) The internship mentioned should be conducted under the supervision of a clinical psychologist who has been practicing for two years, or more
	(3) The internship shall contain total 43 weeks or 1500 h; duration of the practical training mentioned in sub-items (a) to (c) above shall total 9 weeks or 360 h, or more	(3) The number of weeks or hours of internship shall total 48 weeks or 1920 h, or more

Note:[a]The practice items exclusively for clinical psychologists.

primarily the mental health units of hospitals (Lin, 2000; Wang et al., 2011). CPs prefer to say they provide "psychological counselling", while the clinical psychologists and medical doctors prefer to use the term "psychotherapy". Data obtained from the same CPs national survey in Taiwan presented in the first article in this journal issue (Goodyear et al., in press) showing that 57.4% of CPs reported that they perceive themselves to have distinctive differences from the clinical psychologists.

Nevertheless, the Psychologists' Act that bonded the two professionals in one law and defined both of them as medical professionals under the supervision of Ministry of Health and Welfare has blurred the traditional boundaries between the two specialties (Wang et al., 2011). Though very few voices suggested a "one law one profession" approach (Lin & Hsu, 2008); yet, CP and clinical psychology specialties by and by took different roads.

In fact, other than being supervised under the same law and having the same examination date, the two specialties have their own review boards for examination qualifications, boards of examination, test subjects and sets of test items. As the effect of the Act, CP has by and large strengthened its identity and differentiated from clinical psychology through the amendment of requirements for internship programme and national examination subjects. From the content of amendment showed in Table 1, the counselling psychologists have reinforced the normal-developmental professional orientation rather than the psychopathological side of human development.

Post-legislation stage

From the germination of counselling to the birth of the Psychologists' Act, social needs, localized knowledge from the US training systems and strong leading roles of the pioneers in the field have moved CP forward. In this part, we will describe the landscapes of CP in Taiwan in terms of the licensure system, training programmes, professional organizations, employment settings and activities, and opportunities and challenges, which characterize the features of post-legislation stage.

The licensure system in Taiwan

In this part, the national certification examination, internship programme accreditation and quality assurance and continuing education of the licensure system for counselling psychologist are introduced.

National examination for counselling psychologist certification

The national examination for counselling psychologist certification is conducted annually by the Ministry of Examination of Taiwan. Once pass the exam, local health bureaus issue licences on the condition that certified CPs should register in regional counselling psychologists' guilds.

Since 2001, the qualifications for attending the national examination have been amended several times. For example, the Act regulates that, to sit for the examination, a candidate must have a master's degree with a major in CP or related field, finished at least seven specified core areas of coursework and completed an one-year internship. The latest revision has changed the seven core courses into new version beginning on 1 January 2015.

Internship programme accreditation

The quality of internship programme is continuously a major concern for CP leaders. In the first 10 years after the Psychologists' Act, there were no clear accrediting standards for internship programme; so many students chose hospitals as internship sites. However, the supervision received in hospitals that provided by psychiatrists or clinical psychologist in pathological manner had jeopardized the normal-developmental identity of CP (Wang et al., 2011)

With the efforts of academic organizations and professional union, the Psychologists' Act Enforcement Rules was amended to set standards for the internship programme. According to the latest version in 2011, it regulates all internships should be executed consecutively in a qualified institution and be supervised by a qualified counselling psychologist. In addition, the internship should include six areas of activities and comprise at least 43 weeks or 1500 h (see Table 1 for detail information).

The Ministry of Health and Welfare appointed the Taiwan Counselling and Guidance Association (TGCA; formerly CGA) and Taiwan Counselling Psychology Association (TWCPA; founded in 2008 as will be described below) by to accredit internship institutions. TGCA and TWCPA have set criteria collaboratively for the accreditation that began in 2010. The criteria address qualifications of supervisors, supervisor–supervisees ratio, the quantity time of supervision and physical settings. The internship sites could choose either TGCA or TWCPA to be accredited and as of 2014, they together had accredited more than 120 institutions annually (retrieved from http://www.guidance.org.tw/). The websites of the associations have become platforms for interns and institutes seeking or offering internships.

Quality assurance and continuing education

The Psychologists' Act contains specific regulation aimed at protecting the interests of counselling recipients and monitoring the service quality of CPs. For example, two years of professional experience are required to qualify for starting a private clinic and practitioners must protect the privacy of their clients and maintain client records for 10 years. Furthermore, all licenced CPs must receive at least 150 credit hours of continuing education every 6 years in the areas of professional theory and technique, quality assurance, professional ethics and related laws and regulations.

Training institutes

In 1961, Professor Zong Liang-Dung initiated guidance curricula at the Department of Education in National Taiwan Normal University (NTNU) in response to the need for CTs in school systems. The first higher education programme in undergraduate level named "Counselling" was offered in 1971 by Taiwan College of Education (current Department of Counselling and Guidance, National Changhua Normal University, NCNU). Both NTNU and NCNU launched their counselling and guidance graduate programme in 1979. Before the passage of the Psychologists' Act in 2001, there were only eight graduate counselling training programmes. Yet, approximately 28 master's and doctorate level CP programmes now are producing more than 200 certification-eligible graduates each year. The graduate requirements for the master's programmes range from 32 to 45 credit hours and one year of internship experience.

The Psychologists' Act has dramatically transformed Taiwan CP training programmes. Before the Act, CP programmes in different universities varied considerably in focus and curriculum. The effect of licensure has been to standardize the CP curriculum to focus on the seven areas of prerequisites for the National examination, and these have become increasingly specific in response to directives by the Ministry of Examination. With training programmes' unanimously adopting this curriculum, Lin and Hsu's (2008) suggestion of a counselling accreditation organization was not followed.

Other than articulating the course requirements for the National examination, currently, the Enforcement Rules also clearly asserts that a CP programme must contain "Counselling" in its programme's name and force programmes to recruit CP professionals as faculty. As well, TCGA and TWCPA regulate the faculty who served as internship programme advisors must have a CP doctoral degree, at least one year of practical experience in supervision and two years of experience in counselling practice.

Data from the Goodyear's (in press) Taiwan survey showed that 83.9% of the respondents were at the master's level and 16.1% had doctoral degrees. Not reported in that article were additional data showing that 87.9% obtained their degrees in Taiwan, whereas 11.3% obtained their degrees in the US. Respondents were generally satisfied with their choice of CP as a profession ($M = 4.45$ on a five-point scale). Most respondents were satisfied with the quality of theoretical and practical training, internship programmes and supervisors (average of more than 4.00). Only research training was rated lower than 3.5. In addition, 64.5% of respondents reported that internship and supervision was the most helpful part of training, and 20.2% reported that theoretical coursework was the most helpful. The three most frequently suggested coursework were practical experience and supervision (31.4%), cross-profession cooperation training (20.6%) and multicultural counselling training (12.7%).

Main professional organizations

TGCA and TWCPA are the two academic organizations that lead Taiwan's CP development. The Chinese Guidance Association (CGA) changed its name to the Taiwan Guidance and Counselling Association (TGCA) in 2008. Needless to say, CGA played a historical role in Taiwan's CP's development: when TWCPA was formed in 2008 as a spin-off of the CGA's Division of Counselling Psychology, the action shook the identity of TCGA. The TCGA board eventually decided to restore their roles and identity in "guidance and counselling" and to include all members who practiced counselling on diverse settings, particularly in school settings, and with or without licence. Currently, the TGCA has more than 200 group members[2] and 800 individual members (retrieved form http://www.guidance.org.tw/), and continues to be the largest and most influential academic association in Taiwan.

The TWCPA was founded in December 2008 to build up the cooperation between the research and practice of CP, to enhance the identity of CPs, to promote the development of CP specialty and to participate in the related legislation. TWCPA recruits only certified CPs, master's graduates and faculty in the field, which limits their membership numbers (retrieved from http://www.twcpa.org.tw/). Currently, the TWPCA comprises approximately 200 groups and individual members. Although only 10% of practitioners join the TWCPA, the association continues to promote the development of the profession and lead the tide in CP.

The Psychologists' Act requires that all certified CPs must join a regional guild before the local city or country government issues his/her licence, or be fined. The Taipei Counselling Psychologist Association, launched on 1 May 2005, was the first and largest regional guild. The Taiwan Counselling Psychologist Union (TCPU) was founded on 23 January 2010 and represents 12 regional guilds (retrieved from http://www.tcpu.org.tw/). By the end of 2013, the TCPU comprised 2355 members and plays according to the Ministry of Health and Welfare (retrieved from http://www.mohw.gov.tw/).

TGCA, TWCPA and TCPU are the three bellwether organizations that influence the policy and orientation of Taiwan CP's development. Their well cooperation in the past 10 years has created more employment opportunities for the graduates in CP through their active roles in providing the nation's mental health services whenever a trauma event occurred and proactively participating in the legislation process related to mental health issues.

Work settings, typical workdays, theoretical approaches and core values

Results of the Taiwan survey (Goodyear et al., in press) showed that nearly three-fourths (71.7%) of counselling psychologists worked primarily in school settings or for students of all ages, 14.5% worked in social welfare settings, 7.9% worked in private clinics and 2.4% worked in hospitals and medical settings. In addition, the 60% reported that they have secondary work settings.

As mentioned above, Taiwan's CPs adopted normal-developmental and pluralistic theoretic approaches. The top three theoretical approaches that respondents selected were eclectic (38.7%), psychodynamic (16.1%) and Sullivan or interpersonal (8.9%) theories. Respondents reported that their theoretical orientation often influenced their professional practice ($M = 4.11$). Direct services, including psychological assessment, career counselling and consultation, accounted for 61.9% of their time. Furthermore, they devoted an average of 77.8% of their counselling or therapy to individual counselling, 15.3% to group counselling and 13.3% to family counselling.

Four values in the current research were rated more than 4.60 on average, namely "a focus on person – environment interactions" ($M = 4.69$), "attention to people's assets, strengths and resources" ($M = 4.68$), "a focus on developmental issues and developmentally appropriate interventions across the lifespan" ($M = 4.62$) and "a focus on diversity ... in understanding people's experiences" ($M = 4.57$). These results are likely because 70% of CPs work for students and families in schools or related settings, where reflecting the collectivist values of society in Taiwan. Conversely, although doing research is a requisite for pursuing a master's degree in Taiwan, CPs valued "drawing on research to inform practice" ($M = 3.47$) and "producing research that adds to knowledge of counselling psychology-related topics" ($M = 3.65$) the least. It seems that the CPs in Taiwan would prefer "Practitioner" to "Scientist–Practitioner" as their working identity.

Though not reported in Goodyear et al. (in press), it is useful to note that the Taiwan survey revealed that 96.0% of the respondents recognized the importance of personal psychotherapy as a prerequisite for the work of CPs. More than 90% of CPs had personal psychotherapy and satisfied their therapy experience ($M = 3.89$). After being licenced, 88.7% continued to obtain formal supervision; 61.6% were supervised regularly and satisfied with their individual and group supervision quality ($M = 4.22, 3.97$).

Opportunities and challenges

The Psychologists' Act has produced substantial benefits to the CP specialty. First, an increasing number of people are aware of the value of mental health and counselling services have garnered wider societal recognition after the legislation. More employment opportunities were created for the undergraduates or graduates trained by CP, such as court counsellors, specialized school counsellors and CPs in city or county student counselling centres. Second, the professional status of counselling psychologists improved after the legislation in terms of their professional identity and service time. About 75% of respondents identified themselves as practitioners and the percentage of time they reported spending in direct services was 35.3%, an increase from the 26.6% that respondents reported in Lin's (2000) earlier survey of counselling profession. Further, following the social change and urbanization of Taiwan, most respondents regarded this trend as a promising opportunity for CPs.

However, respondents to our survey identified three major challenges. First, counselling services provided by CPs are not covered by the National Health Insurance or any other private insurance.[3] People who require mental health services are reluctant or unable to pay for such services, which impedes the development of counselling

industries. Second, the over-expanding of university counselling psychology programmes after legislation could endanger training quality and crowd the job market.

The third challenge arises from the profession itself. The need for counselling services is increasing but the service qualities are uneven. The ecological counselling
approach that emphasizes on working with family and school systems is increasingly a
significant approach since more than 70% of CPs work in school settings. But CP training in Taiwan still is mainly oblique to the assessment and counselling of individuals
(Wang et al., 2008).

Given the influence of Western theories of counselling psychotherapy in Taiwan's
CP training models, the localization of CP in Taiwan's social and culture context is perceived as an indispensable challenge to the professionals of vision. An appeal for promoting the counselling research of Chinese culture-inclusion was first launched by the
editor in chief of *Taiwan Counselling Quarterly* (Wang, 2013). A website for the academic community of indigenous counselling was constructed (http://ic.heart.net.tw/),
and a special column for the issue of Chinese indigenous counselling was generated
(Wang, 2014). Apart from that, the subject of "Research and Practice of Indigenous
Counselling" was a main theme of the 2014 TGCA annual conference. In recent years,
more and more creative healing approach, research and practices have developed and
applied indigenously (Chen, 2009; Jin, 2005; Liu et al., 2014). Among those studies,
Jin (2005) has promoted an expressive healing method named "the psychological displacement paradigm of diary writing (PDPD)" that merged the concept derived from
Chinese Philosophy and Western CP theories has gained evidence-based recognition in
the field (Chang et al., 2013; Jin, 2010; Lee & Jin, in press; Seih et al., 2008; Wang
et al., 2012).

It is our anticipation to promote CP as a unique specialty that possesses Taiwan's
characteristics and features fitting into our society; nevertheless, it is continuing to be
the challenges and responsibilities of Taiwan's CP professionals.

Disclosure statement

No potential conflict of interest was reported by the authors.

Notes

1. The Student Guidance and Counselling Act was promulgated on 12 November 2014.
2. Group members are comprised of member organizations, such as schools, counselling centres,
   university departments, associations and other organizations related to the specialty.
3. The psychotherapies conducted by medial doctors and clinical psychologists in hospital or
   medical settings are covered by the National Health Insurance.

References

Chang, J. H., Huang, C. L., & Lin, Y. C. (2013). The psychological displacement paradigm in diary-writing (PDPD) and its psychological benefits. *Journal of Happiness Studies, 14*, 155–167.

Chen, P. (2009). A counselling model for self-relation coordination for Chinese client with interpersonal conflicts. *The Counseling Psychologist, 37*, 987–1009.

Goodyear, R. K., Lichtenberg, J. W., Hutman, H., Overland, E., Bedi, R., Christiani, K., & Young, C. (in press). A global portrait of counselling psychologists' characteristics, perspectives, and professional behaviors. *Counselling Psychology Quarterly.* doi: 10.1080/09515070.2015.1128396.

Hsiao, W., & Jin, S. (1996). *"The standards for professional counselors' work level and qualification" project.* Taipei, Taiwan: Educational Commissioners of Educational Bureau.

Jin, S. R. (2005). *The dialectical effect of psychological displacement: A narrative analysis.* Taipei: National Science Council.

Jin, S. R. (2010). Structure characteristics of psychological displacement and its dialectical phenomenon: Narratives of the multidimensional self. *Chinese Journal of Guidance and Counselling, 28*, 191–233.

Lee, F., & Jin, S. R. (in press). Research on the words structure and connotation of psychological displacement paradigm in diary-writing (PDPD): A discourse analysis. *Journal of Educational Psychology.*

Lin, C. (2000). The preference identity, work settings, and service hours of mental health professionals – A comparison study. *Journal of Educational Psychology, 32*(1), 1–14.

Lin, C., & Hsu, H. (2008). The legislation impacts of the psychologists' Act. *Guidance Quarterly, 44*, 24–33.

Liu, S. H., Wang, C. H., Deng, C. P., Keh, F. B., Lu, Y. J., & Tsai, Y. C. (2014). Action research using a Chinese career model based on the wisdom of classic of changes and its applications. *Journal of Pacific Rim Psychology, 8*, 83–94.

Seih, Y. T., Lin, Y. C., Huang, C. L., Peng, C. W., & Huang, S. P. (2008). The benefits of psychological displacement in diary writing when using different pronouns. *British Journal of Health Psychology, 13*, 39–41.

The Counselling Psychologists' Act (R.O.C. Const. 2001).

The Counselling Psychologists' Act Enforcement Rules (R.O.C. Const. 2011 amendment).

The Professional and Technologists Psychologists Examination Rules (R.O.C. Const. 2013 amendment).

Wang, C. H. (2013). Crossing the nations: Promoting the counselling research of Chinese culture-inclusion. *Taiwan Counselling Quarterly, 5*, vi.

Wang, C. H. (2014). Based on Chinese culture, contribution to universal counselling: The founding of Chinese academic community of indigenous counselling and the establishment of column of Chinese indigenous counselling. *Taiwan Counselling Quarterly, 6*, vi–ix.

Wang, L., Kwan, K. K., & Huang, S. (2011). Counselling psychology licensure in Taiwan: Development, challenges, and opportunities. *International Journal for the Advancement of Counselling, 33*, 37–50.

Wang, Y. L., Lin, Y. C., Huang, C. L., & Yeh, K. H. (2012). Benefitting from a different perspective: The effect of a complementary matching of psychological distance and habitual perspective on emotion regulation. *Asian Journal of Social Psychology, 15*, 198–207.

Wang, L., Tu, S., & Chao, H. (2008). An exploratory investigation of effective counselling strategies for counselling psychologists working in elementary schools. *Bulletin of Educational Psychology, 39*, 413–434.

Yeh, I. (2013). *The developmental history of Taiwan school guidance.* Taipei: Psychology Publishing.

Counselling psychology in the United Kingdom

Jessica D. Jones Nielsen[a] and Helen Nicholas[b]

[a]Department of Psychology, City University London, London, UK; [b]Department of Psychology, University of Worcester, Worcestershire, UK

Counselling psychology within the UK has grown over the last three decades, adapting to many changes in the field of applied psychology, whilst remaining true to its core values and humanistic origins. The identity of counselling psychology is strongly rooted in a relational stance and applied psychology, where attention to psychological formulation is given to improve psychological functioning and well-being. This article outlines a brief history of counselling psychology in the UK, the training process, credentialing and looks at some important challenges and future directions for counselling psychology in the UK. A proportion of the members from the British Psychological Society's division of counselling psychology (DCoP, $N = 148$) took part in the study. Participants provided demographic, training, employment, workplace and career pathway information obtained through an online questionnaire distributed to all DCoP members. On the whole, DCoP members are working in a variety of areas within the UK and the findings of this article contribute to the international study comparing counselling psychology across the globe.

Brief history of counselling psychology in the UK

Counselling psychology became recognised as a specialty in the UK when the British Psychological Society (BPS) established the Counselling Psychology Section in 1982. The establishment of this section arose out of the need to consider the relationship between psychology and counselling in the UK, and recognise counselling psychology's status in the applied psychology field. In 1989, the Section became a "Special Group," with its own practice guidelines and served as a "half-way house" between a scientific interest group and a professional body (Strawbridge & Woolfe, 2003). The creation of the Special Group provided the structure and establishment of the Diploma in Counselling which was a formally recognized route to Chartered Status for professionals wishing to specialise in counselling psychology. By 1994, after much work to launch the professional status of counselling psychology within the BPS and wider society, the Special Group was given the status of a full division within the BPS (Corrie & Callahan, 2000). Indeed, in the space of three decades, counselling psychology has established itself as a full specialty of applied psychologists in the UK alongside the other applied psychology divisions such as clinical, occupational and educational.

The Division of Counselling Psychology (DCoP) has continued to grow in status and in membership, and aims to promote the professional interests of counselling psychologists as well as to develop psychology as a profession and as a body of knowledge and skills. There are currently over 3,500 members in the DCoP, and many members are actively involved within the BPS boards. The Division also has branches in Northern Ireland, Scotland and Wales for members in these areas. The Branch chairs are members of and report to the DCoP executive committee. The DCoP publishes a quarterly, peer-reviewed journal, *the Counselling Psychology Review*, which is distributed free of charge to members. The journal focuses on high-quality research pertinent to the work of counselling psychologists both in the UK and internationally. Our members also enjoy benefits of the Society, which include support from professional groups and networks, a monthly copy of the BPS in-house magazine, *The Psychologist*, access to job advertisements, journals, conference attendance and discounts on books.

Credentialing

All counselling psychologists are regulated by the Health and Care Professions Council (HCPC) which has set the threshold for qualification at doctoral level (or equivalent) since 2009. The HCPC is a regulatory body set up under the authority of Parliament to protect the public by maintaining a register for 16 health and care professions which include practitioner psychologists. It is a requirement for professionals working in these roles to be registered with the HCPC. The title of "Counselling Psychologist" is one of the protected titles under the practitioner psychologist profession alongside the following eight titles: Clinical Psychologist, Educational Psychologist, Forensic Psychologist, Health Psychologist, Occupational Psychologist, Practitioner Psychologist, Registered Psychologist, and Sport and Exercise Psychologist. The Standards of Proficiency (SOP) for practitioner psychologists list both generic standards as well as more profession-specific standards. Counselling psychologists are required to register with the HCPC and undertake to meet the SOP set out by the HCPC in order to practice "lawfully, safely and effectively" (HCPC, 2012b). The HCPC also publishes standards of conduct, performance and ethics (HCPC, 2012a). In order to be registered to practice, psychologists in the UK need to earn a qualification from an HCPC-approved programme, and demonstrate that they have met the standards set forth by the HCPC. The BPS role in terms of regulation has been to work with the HCPC to promote the specialty, represent members, curriculum frameworks, post-registration education and training, and continuing professional development.

The BPS is the representative body for psychology and psychologists in the UK. It was granted its Royal Charter in 1965. The Society has national responsibility for the development, promotion and application of psychology for the public good, and promotes the efficiency and usefulness of its members by maintaining a high standard of professional education and knowledge. The title "Chartered Psychologist" is legally recognised under the Royal Charter. Those who the Society has deemed eligible to do so are entitled to use the designation "Chartered Psychologist" and the abbreviation *CPsychol* after their name.

In order to become chartered, a psychologist must be a member of the BPS and have: (a) achieved a first degree in psychology recognized by the Society as meeting the Graduate Basis for Chartered Membership, (b) undertaken Society accredited post graduate qualifications and training, and (c) agreed to follow the Society's Member Conduct Rules and be guided by the Society's Code of Ethics and Conduct. By adhering to the BPS Membership Conduct Rules and Code of Ethics and Conduct, Chartered Psychologists demonstrate to their clients, who may include patients, students, research participants, educational institutions or organisations, that they uphold the highest levels of professional standards and ethics (BPS, 2009).

Where do counselling psychologists work

Counselling psychologists have become a growing presence in a variety of settings throughout the UK including hospitals (acute admissions, psychiatric intensive care, rehabilitation), health centres, Improving Access to Psychological Therapy (IAPT) Services, Community Mental Health Teams and Child and Adolescent Mental Health Services. They also work within private hospitals, private practice, forensic settings, industry, education, research, and corporate institutions.

It is instructive to examine the results of the recent survey of UK counselling psychology, many of which are summarised in the article that introduces this issue of the CPQ (Goodyear et al., in press). The sample was representative of the DCOP in terms of age (33%, 51–65 years), gender (73% female), ethnicity (95% White) and membership status (48% Chartered Member, 49% Associate Fellow and 3% Fellow).

Career pathway and current employment

Table 3 in Goodyear et al. (in press) indicates that nearly a third (32%) of respondents are currently working with the National Health Service (NHS). In addition to the NHS, there are other work-setting categories that were more specific to the UK and not reported in Table 3. Those settings and their percentages are therefore reported in Table 1 below. It shows, for example, that 29.5% reported working in private practice ($N = 25$) or were self-employed ($N = 13$). A further 10.8% ($N = 11$ and $N = 3$) were working within university counselling centres and university departments, respectively. Seven percent ($N = 9$) indicated they were working in medical settings outside of the NHS including forensic services, general hospitals, psychiatric hospitals, primary and secondary care settings. As well – and also in more specific set of categories than were used in Goodyear et al. – 49% of respondents identified as clinical practitioners ($N = 72$), 10% as consultants ($N = 15$) and 11% as either directors ($N = 6$), head of services ($N = 6$) or clinical leads ($N = 4$) for their primary professional roles. Of those in academic posts, 2 (18%) were appointed on the professorial scale, 9% ($N = 1$) as Reader, 36% ($N = 4$) as Senior Lecturers and 27% ($N = 3$) as Lecturer.

With regards to professional activities, a large proportion of respondents reported they were providing psychological counselling/psychotherapy (20%) and clinical intervention (13%). The proportion of respondents who reported engagement in either administration/management, clinical assessment/formulation, assessment, clinical supervision and teaching/training at 10, 10, 9, 8 and 6%, respectively. Of the respondents who indicated providing psychological counselling/psychotherapy, indicated that a large

Table 1. Primary work settings of counselling psychologists in the UK.

	N	%
NHS	41	31.8
Private practice	25	19.4
Self-employed	13	10.1
Private sector	12	9.3
University department	11	8.5
Non profit/Voluntary sector	7	5.4
Public sector	3	2.3
Primary care	3	2.3
University counselling centres	3	2.3
Other (please specify)	3	2.3
Forensic services and prisons	2	1.6
General health/hospital settings	2	1.6
Professional school of psychology	2	1.6
Secondary care	1	.8
Psychiatric hospital/centre	1	.8
Total	129	

proportion of their time was dedicated to practising individual psychological counselling/psychotherapy out of the following five types of counselling interventions: individual (33%), couples (26%), group (26%), family (10%) and organisational (6%).

Main professional counselling psychology organisations in the UK

There are various professional counselling psychology-related organisations in the UK. However, the main professional counselling and psychotherapy bodies that have taken on the role of self-regulation of counselling/psychotherapy include: British Association for Counselling and Psychotherapy (BACP), Counselling & Psychotherapy in Scotland (COSCA), Health and Care Professions Council (HCPC), Irish Association for Counselling and Psychotherapy (IACP), the National Counselling Society (NCS) and the United Kingdom Council for Psychotherapy (UKCP). Of course the list of professional organisations is not exhaustive, but the ones listed are those that have a substantial presence of counselling psychologists represented within each organisation.

Training in counselling psychology

Training in counselling psychology is through a BPS accredited doctoral programme. As of 2015, 13 university institutions are offering the Counselling Psychology doctorate: City University, University of East London, Glasgow Caledonian University, London Metropolitan University, University of Manchester, Metanoia Institute (London), New School of Psychotherapy & Counselling (London), Regent's University London, University of Roehampton, University of Surrey, University of Teesside, University of the West of England, and University of Wolverhampton. The Qualification in Counselling Psychology (QCoP), also known as the independent route, is regulated and offered by the BPS and upon successful completion of the QCoP candidates are eligible to apply for Chartered Membership and to apply to the HCPC for registration as a counselling psychologist. Candidates applying to train through this route are not attached to a particular university, choosing to study independently, designing their own work-place based learning and submitting assignments linked to criteria of competencies. This flexibility is advantageous given that counselling psychologists in the UK pay for their university education and enables the candidates to gain the necessary work experience whilst training. Along with the flexibility of the independent route, candidates need to take responsibility for designing, organising and arranging their training programme, supervision, placements and resources. The QCoP is overseen by the Counselling Psychology Qualifications Board who is accountable to the Qualifications Standards Committee, reporting to the membership Standards Board and ultimately to the BPS Board of Trustees. For further information regarding the enrolment requirements please see the *Qualification in Counselling Psychology Enrolment Guidelines* (2014b).

The BPS has been involved in the accreditation of programmes of education and training in psychology since the early 1970s (BPS, 2014a). The Society accredits programmes at both undergraduate (and equivalent) and postgraduate levels. Undergraduate, conversion and integrated Masters programmes are accredited against the requirements for the Society's Graduate Basis for Chartered (GBC) membership, the curriculum requirements for which are derived from the Quality Assurance Agency's Subject Benchmark Statement for Psychology. Postgraduate programmes are accredited against the knowledge, practice and research requirements for Chartered Psychologist (CPsychol) status in a range of domains of practice (BPS, 2010). A number of the postgraduate programmes that are accredited by the Society are also approved by the HCPC, the statutory regulator of practitioner psychologists in the UK.

In order to ensure that quality standards in psychology education and training are met by all programmes, the BPS works collaboratively with education providers using the Accreditation through Partnership process. Accreditation through Partnership is a model that focuses on promoting psychology as a science, and on the development of transferable skills to enhance graduate employability. It promotes a spirit of supportive enquiry, rather than prescribing a particular approach to student development or programme delivery. The Society publishes standards for the accreditation of undergraduate, conversion and integrated masters programmes in psychology, and for postgraduate programmes of professional training. The BPS postgraduate standards span eight domains of practice, seven of which relate to pre-qualification training leading to Chartered Membership of the Society, and full membership of one or more of the Society's Divisions (the Division of Clinical Psychology, the Division of Counselling Psychology, the Division of Educational and Child Psychology or the Scottish Division of Educational Psychology, the Division of Forensic Psychology, the Division of Health Psychology, the Division of Occupational Psychology and the Division of Sport and Exercise Psychology). These correspond to the seven protected titles regulated by the HCPC.

Counselling psychology in comparison to other closely related specialties in the UK

Unlike counselling and psychotherapy which developed separately outside of the profession of psychology, counselling psychology in the UK, concerns itself with the development and evaluation of practice and attention to the relationship (Strawbridge & Woolfe, 2003). Furthermore, counselling psychology has benefitted from a breadth of overlap with other applied psychology specialties, including clinical psychology (Strawbridge & Woolfe, 2010). However, when attempting to characterise counselling psychology, comparisons are often drawn from what separates it from other specialities (Walsh & Frankland, 2009). With a strong focus on the therapeutic relationship, counselling psychology adheres to the scientist–practitioner model of professional practice (Corrie & Callahan, 2000), and the reflective practitioner model (Schon, 1983). In the UK, counselling psychologists are well-represented across a variety of mental health settings and are well-regarded within allied mental health disciplines. Counselling psychologists, in particular, have enjoyed interdisciplinary team working with other allied mental health professionals across a variety of settings and with its unique ability to position itself alongside other specialties that champion the scientist–practitioner model.

Similar to other countries, it is becoming more difficult to differentiate counselling psychologists from clinical psychologists in the UK as they are both part of the applied psychology field. Both professions operate from within the scientist–practitioner model and emphasize evidence-based practice. Applied psychologist often compete for similar jobs in the NHS, and have comparable skills sets in being able to provide treatment, assessment and consultation. However, counselling psychologists in the UK are committed to exploring a range of approaches of psychology which include existential and humanistic, psychoanalytic/psychodynamic and cognitive-behavioural. The latter approach is often the emphasis of clinical psychologists in science and practice along with the biomedical model.

Within the UK, clinical psychology training is funded through the NHS as well as clinical psychology trainees being salaried members of NHS staff, whilst undergoing their doctoral training. There are currently 30 training courses in the UK offering the clinical psychology doctoral training compared to the 14 courses (including the independent route) offering counselling psychology doctorate courses.

Core values of counselling psychologists in the UK

Counselling psychology in the UK holds a humanistic value base with influences from counselling psychology in the USA and European psychotherapy. With a focus on the application of psychological and psychotherapeutic theory and to clinical practice, the science of psychology remains important within our field (British Psychological Society Division of Counselling Psychology, 2012). According to the standards for counselling psychology, the aim of counselling psychology is to reduce psychological distress and to promote the well-being of individuals by focusing on their subjective experience as it unfolds in their interaction with the physical, social, cultural and spiritual dimensions in living. Counselling psychology also places relational practice at its centre, and therefore, the therapeutic relationship is considered to be the main vehicle through which psychological difficulties are understood and alleviated. As an applied area of psychology, counselling psychology in the UK is a specific discipline that is concerned with the study of being (ontology), the nature of "how we know what we know" (epistemology) and praxis (clinical application). In its concern with philosophy, counselling psychology embraces a pluralistic and interdisciplinary attitude which overlaps with other applied psychologies, counselling, psychotherapy, psychiatry, and the political and economic systems that sustain them.

"At the centre of counselling psychology lies an inquisitive, reflexive and critical attitude that acknowledges the diversity of ontological and epistemological positions underlying all forms of therapeutic approaches and techniques. It is a stance that holds a humanistic and relational value system which aims at the exploration, clarification and understanding of clients' world-views, underlying assumptions and emotional difficulties that emerge out of our interaction with the world and others. In line with the above philosophical thinking and praxis, counselling psychologists' distinctive identity is reflected in their high levels of competence to work both with structure/content and with process/interpersonal dynamics as they unfold during the therapeutic encounter. Moreover, they bring aspects of themselves to their work, derived from their training, wider knowledge, and lived experience. In contrast to the medical model, assessment, formulation of emotional and relational difficulties in living, and therapeutic plan are seen as parts of an inherently relational and shared enterprise that is informed both by professional expertise and the uniqueness of the human encounter between practitioner and client. It is a therapeutic endeavour that distinguishes the field from other applied psychologies by its explicit use of a phenomenological and hermeneutic inquiry that enhances the aforementioned inquisitive, reflexive, and critical attitude when engaging with medical, psychopharmacological, and classification literature as well as use of nomothetic (psychometric and neurological) testing" (pp. 15–16).

Challenges facing counselling psychologist in the UK

One of the main challenges facing UK applied psychologists is employment and employability. More than half of the Division's membership works in the NHS and with the many structural changes our members and applied psychologists in general are facing increasing pressure. This pressure is coming from a need to deliver effective treatment services with more emphasis on cost. As a result, positions are being downgraded and there is increased competition between applied psychologists for limited roles. The increased demand for services to provide effective treatment, in some cases, has led services to rely more on "cheaper" alternatives, such as psychological well-being practitioners and other less-qualified individuals, as well as an increase in online counselling and self-study. Applied psychologists are therefore forced into an environment where raising their profile and differentiating psychology in the eyes of commissioners and service managers becomes vital.

Counselling psychologists are strongly represented, for example, in independent practice, forensics, academic, and third sectors. More recently, they are increasingly working in partnership across sectors and bidding for public work using different organisational frameworks. A recent publication "An Introduction to Bidding for Public Sector Contracts for Counselling Psychologists" (Vermes, 2013) was written to meet this demand. The publication provides psychologists working in small independent services an overview of the steps necessary to prepare to bid for and deliver services under contract to the NHS and its local trusts, and other public mental health commissioning bodies such as local authorities. Maintaining a strong representation of counselling psychology in the NHS is beneficial in terms of professional standing and public/professional awareness of the specialty. The benefits of increasing our cross-divisional working and work with other applied psychologists may raise concerns for members who want to maintain their identity as counselling psychologists. This challenge of maintaining our identity and ensuring we gain equity of employment is a challenge that will continue to face counselling psychologists.

The BPS, through member networks, identifies expertise when responding to government consultations and other organisations. The challenge for counselling psychologists is to access workforce and membership data to enable us to gain the volunteer workforce to be involved in these projects. Counselling psychologists maintain key positions on the BPS's boards, working groups and projects where we can influence policy and practice for counselling psychologists. Currently, our membership and workforce data is not effective enough to allow us to access our membership sufficiently. The DCoP is reliant on a voluntary workforce and the difficulties with recruiting volunteers onto the divisional committee has been challenging in the past. This workforce and membership data is vital and is needed to determine the areas of specialism critical to meeting the demands of consultations, mentoring, leadership and supervision.

The regulation of practitioner psychologists has been in the hands of the HCPC since 2009. Since then the title "practitioner psychologist" has been protected along with clinical psychologist, counselling psychologist, educational psychologist, forensic psychologist, health psychologist, occupational psychologist, sport and exercise psychologist. The HCPC did not protect the title "psychologist." This omission has raised some concerns that individuals who do not meet the requirements for registration under one of the statutory protected titles describe themselves by using the term "psychologist" which may lead the public to believe they are delivering the services of a psychologist. Applied psychologists have been encouraged to use the HCPC logo and their registration number on documents and to raise any concerns with the HCPC to investigate.

The future of counselling psychology in the UK

The DCoP continues to grow in number and in strength and has played a vital part in a number of key policy changes within the BPS, the field of counselling psychology and government. This has proved valuable in meeting the increased demands from consultation from e.g. Government, the Department of Health, Public Health England, NICE, the various mental health alliances of which the BPS is a member and also internal Society documents prior to issue.

Addressing the employment and employability challenge has highlighted the competencies, unique identity and valuable contribution that counselling psychologists can bring to the workforce. As counselling psychologists continue to expand into employment and practice areas, independent practice, utilizing their unique values and abilities, providing quality continuing development training and developing their own areas of specialism, our workforce is more able to meet the needs of the increasing demands on services. The flexibility that the counselling psychology doctoral training provides our trainees will ensure that our members are widely skilled in a variety of key areas. This will help us meet the challenges facing us and grow from the opportunities and struggles that may arise in the years to come.

The Division has continued to make valuable connections with international colleagues within a number of APA divisions, including taking part in this international survey. We have also developed stronger ties with other applied psychologists, BPS Divisions, Sections and Branches as well as with related specialities. Our attention to an increase in outwardly focused research, showcasing the work of counselling psychologists at our annual conferences and in our journal, will continue to highlight our specialty and provide us with the resources to meet the changes that are presented in future.

The various Network and Interest Groups include a wide range of areas that are of particular interest to members of the DCoP and to other applied psychologists. These include groups on social justice, NHS, Black and Asian counselling psychologist group, spirituality, Dementia, children and young adults, learning disability, palliative care, counselling psychologists working in forensic settings and a group for counselling psychologists working within "Improving Access to Psychological Therapy" (IAPT) group, a primary care setting.

The need for services is increasing and the cost of mental health services does require the government to think about smarter investments in early interventions and prevention. There is a general governmental shift towards more focus on person-centred care, a value held firmly by counselling psychologists since it began. The need for clients to have a genuine choice when it comes to therapeutic interventions is best suited to counselling psychologists and their diversity. This opens up a range of opportunities for us to contribute in a unique way to services and to multispecialist centres. The future for counselling psychology and counselling psychologists is ever changing, however, we have the competencies, flexibility and knowledge to move with the times, to adjust and adapt whilst maintaining our unique identity within the applied psychology field.

Key articles and other sources regarding counselling psychology in the UK

Many of the publications cited in this article provide useful information about counselling psychology in the UK, but for readers who desire a couple of especially comprehensive reviews of the specialty, we would recommend Woolfe, Dryden, and Strawbridge (2009) as well as Woolfe (2012).

Disclosure statement

No potential conflict of interest was reported by the authors.

References

British Psychological Society. (2009). *Code of ethics and conduct*. Leicester: BPS.

British Psychological Society Division of Counselling Psychology. (2010). *Guidance for counselling psychology programmes*. Leicester: BPS.

British Psychological Society Division of Counselling Psychology. (2012). *Becoming a counselling psychologist*. Retrieved from http:www.bps.org.uk/dcop/home/about/about_home.cfm

British Psychological Society Division of Counselling Psychology. (2014a). *Standards for the accreditation of doctoral programmes in counselling psychology*. Leicester: Author.

British Psychological Society Division of Counselling Psychology. (2014b). *Qualification in counselling psychology enrolment guidelines*. Retrieved from http://www.bps.org.uk/system/files/Public%20files/Quals/enrolment_guidelines.pdf

Corrie, S., & Callahan, M. (2000). A review of the scientist-practitioner model: Reflections on its potential contribution to counselling psychology within the context of current healthcare trends. *British Journal of Medical Psychology*. Sep; 73 (Pt3), 413–427.

Goodyear, R. K., Lichtenberg, J. W., Hutman, H., Overland, E., Bedi, R., Christiani, K., … Young, C. (in press). A global portrait of counselling psychologists' characteristics, perspectives, and professional behaviors. *Counselling Psychology Quarterly*. doi:10.1080/09515070.2015.1128396

Health and Care Professions Council. (2012a). *Standards of conduct, performance and ethics*. Retrieved from http://www.hpc-uk.org/assets/documents/10003B6EStandardsofconduct,performanceandethics.pdf

Health and Care Professions Council. (2012b). *Standards of proficiency: Practitioner psychologists*. Retrieved from http://www.hcpc-uk.org/assets/documents/10002963SOP_Practitioner_psychologists.pdf

Schon, D. (1983). *The reflective practitioner: How professionals think in action*. New York, NY: Basic Books.

Strawbridge, S., & Woolfe, R. (2003). Counselling psychology in context. In R. Woolfe, W. Dryden, & S. Strawbridge (Eds.), *Handbook of counselling psychology* (2nd ed., pp. 3–22). London: Sage.

Strawbridge, S., & Woolfe, R. (2010). Counselling psychology: Origins, developments and challenges. In R. Woolfe, S. Strawbridge, B. Douglas, & W. Dryden (Eds.), *Handbook of counselling psychology* (3rd ed., pp. 3–22). London: Sage.

Vermes, C. (2013). *An introduction to bidding for public sector contracts for counselling psychologists*. Leicester: BPS.

Walsh, Y., & Frankland, A. (2009). The next 10 years: Some reflections on earlier predictions for counselling psychology. *Counselling Psychology Review, 24*, 38–43.

Woolfe, R. (2012). Risorgimento: A history of counselling psychology in Britain. *Counselling Psychology Review, 27*, 72–78.

Woolfe, R., Dryden, W., & Strawbridge, S. (Eds.). (2009). *Handbook of counselling psychology* (3rd ed.). London: Sage.

Counselling psychology in the United States

James W. Lichtenberg[a], Rodney K. Goodyear[b], Heidi Hutman[c] and
Emily A. Overland[a]

[a]*Department of Educational Psychology, University of Kansas, Lawrence, KS, USA;* [b]*Graduate
Department of Leadership and Counseling, University of Redlands, Redlands, CA, USA;*
[c]*Division of Counseling Psychology, University at Albany, State University of New York, Albany,
NY, USA*

Counseling psychology (CP) emerged in the US as the result of the convergence
of a number of trends in early applied psychology, a number of social factors, as
well as changes in the organizational structure of the American Psychological
Association. We offer an overview of the history of counseling psychology in
the US, focusing on key events that have helped establish and shape the profession. Struggles over the definition of CP as a specialty and its relations with clinical psychology and professional counseling are discussed, as are matters related
to the licensing of CP practitioners, and the profession's relationships with coun-
seling-related professional organizations. The educational and professional
preparation of CPs, the profession's core values that affect both training in and
the practice of counseling psychology, and the settings in which CPs work are
briefly described. We close with a discussion of several of the challenges facing
CP as it is organized and institutionalized in the US.

This paper describes counseling psychology (CP) in the United States (US), with
attention to how country-specific factors and trends have influenced the discipline. It
begins with a review of how the specialty evolved in the US, including key historical
events that led to its emergence. It then addresses some of the issues that continue to
shape the nature and scope of CP in its US context.

History of CP in the US

Founded in 1892 by Dr. G. Stanley Hall, the American Psychological Association
(APA) was established to represent what was then the new and developing field of psychology. As that field developed as a scientific discipline, so did its applications –
including those clinical applications of "the new psychology." Over time, the applied
and clinical members of the association grew dissatisfied with the APA, believing that it

failed to provide an outlet for discussions of professional practice. Instead, these meetings were devoted exclusively to the presentation of scientific papers. Accordingly, in 1937, the clinical practitioners and other applied psychologists within and outside of the APA, branched off and formed the separate American Association of Applied Psychology (AAAP; Munley, Duncan, Mcdonnell, & Sauer, 2004).

However, the absence of a single unifying organization for psychologists became problematic during World War II, particularly with respect to the accompanying efforts to coordinate psychological services in the US. In response, the AAAP and APA merged into a single professional organization in late 1945 (Dewsbury, 1999). The resulting association was organized around an increasingly diffuse conceptualization of psychology – one encompassing the professional practice psychology and the promotion of human welfare, as well as the study and advancement of psychology as a science.

This diffusion of psychology was reflected in APA's divisional structure. In it, members could join interest groups (or sections) in which they could find others with whom they shared common professional interests. APA approved 19 initial divisions in 1944, with the two largest being clinical psychology and personnel guidance psychology. The latter established itself as the Division of Counseling and Guidance – which later became the Division of Counseling Psychology (Gelso, Williams, & Fretz, 2014).

With the end of World War II, the mental health, educational, and vocational concerns of returning veterans brought about a large infusion of federal financial support for the university training of clinical and personnel-related psychologists. This period was especially formative for CP. Prior to the war, mental health treatments generally were provided by psychiatrists and by social workers working under their supervision. But the war created shortages in these personnel that allowed psychologists to begin offering services.

To this end, the Veterans Administration (VA) was formed after the war to serve the millions of returning veterans, and because both counseling and clinical psychologists were placed in VA settings during their training, the VA was heavily involved in and significantly shaped the training and work functions of psychologists (see, Albee, 1998). Moreover, most university counseling centers were established to serve the many returning veterans who became students (Heppner & Neal, 1983) during this period. Given that many CPs worked in university counseling centers, WWII and the return of veterans postwar played a uniquely important role in the history of the discipline.

In August, 1951, following the lead of Division 12 (Clinical Psychology) which, at a conference in Boulder, CO (the "Boulder Conference;" Raimy, 1950), developed training standards for clinical psychology, Division 17 (Counseling and Guidance), sponsored a Conference on the Training of Counseling Psychologists at Northwestern University. The terms "counselling psychology" and "counselling psychologist" were introduced for the first time at that conference (Super, 1955). Conference participants also articulated the roles and functions of CPs, recommended that CPs be trained at the doctoral level, made recommendations concerning practicum and research training, along with core content areas of study for the doctorate in counseling psychology (American Psychological Association [APA], 1952a, 1952b), and initiated the Division 17 name change to the Division of Counseling Psychology.

The initial report from this conference (APA, 1952a) recommended that CP graduate training include basic core knowledge expected of all psychologists and emphasized that research training was essential. The report's emphasis on *both* science and practice in training joined what clinical psychology had previously articulated as the Scientist–Practitioner Model of graduate training (also known as the "Boulder Model;" see Raimy, 1950). In that same year, 1951, the US VA created the job title of counseling psychologist (in two versions: "Vocational" and "Vocational Rehabilitation and Education") for which it required the same levels of training as for clinical psychologists (Blocher, 2000).

Subsequent national training conferences have further articulated training standards for CP. The two most notable being the Greyston Conference held at Columbia University (Thompson & Super, 1964) and the Atlanta Conference (Weissberg et al., 1988).

CP definition

The Division of Counseling Psychology Committee on Definition developed an initial formal definition of CP (APA, 1956). That definition was further delineated in 1981, when the APA published its Specialty Guidelines for the Delivery of Services by Counseling Psychologists (APA, 1981). Subsequent definitions and descriptions have been developed as the specialty evolved. The most recent archival description, which was prepared for CP by APA's Commission on the Recognition of Specialties and Proficiencies in Professional Psychology (CRSPPP), the body within APA that is responsible for validating the existence of current and emerging new specialties in applied psychology, was published online by the APA in 2013 (http://www.apa.org/ed/graduate/special ize/counseling.aspx). That description defines CP as

> ... a general practice and health service provider specialty in professional psychology. It focuses on how people function both personally and in their relationships at all ages. Counseling psychology addresses the emotional, social, work, school and physical health concerns people may have at different stages in their lives, focusing on typical life stresses and more severe issues with which people may struggle as individuals and as a part of families, groups and organizations. Counseling psychologists help people with physical, emotional and mental health issues improve their sense of well-being, alleviate feelings of distress and resolve crises. They also provide assessment, diagnosis, and treatment of more severe psychological symptoms. (retrieved 24 August 2015)

Counseling psychology as a distinct specialty

CP's distinctiveness as an applied psychological specialty, especially its ability to define itself as distinctive from clinical psychology and counseling, has been an issue since CP's early years (Gelso et al., 2014). Reflecting the longstanding nature of this issue, Weigel (1977), writing before the adoption of CSPPP's specialty recognition criteria forced a differentiation from clinical psychology, noted tongue in cheek that CPs were in the bind of wanting "to be neither fish (fish are clinical psychologists: they are cold fish who believe in the medical model ...) nor foul (foul are counselor educators and guidance and counseling graduates ...)" (p. 51).

So how does CP distinguish itself from counseling, from guidance, from personnel psychology, and from clinical psychology? These fields share a number of historical threads and contemporary overlaps, but especially relevant to APA's recognition of specialties is the question of whether CP can be distinguished from other applied psychological specialties in terms of its specialized knowledge, the sorts of problems the profession addresses, the skills and procedures used by the profession, and the population(s) served – CRSPPP's criteria for distinguishing specialties in applied psychology. CP's distinctiveness from clinical psychology has been critical, but at times difficult, to establish. Indeed, as Blocher (2000) noted, in 1959, the Education and Training Board of the APA considered eliminating CP as a recognized distinctive specialty and combining it with clinical psychology.

In this regard, at the time of the initial implementation of CRSPPP's role in recognizing specialties within professional psychology, there was some sense that the only individuals truly interested in and able to find a distinction between clinical and counseling psychology were the faculty in those training programs; because without a purported distinction, universities housing both programs would reasonably close one of the programs or combine them into a single program – likely a clinical psychology program. CP's ongoing efforts to differentiate itself from clinical psychology are reflected in its inclusion of a statement on "What is the difference between a clinical psychologist and a counseling psychologist?" on the SCP webpage (http://www.div17.org/about-cp/counseling-vs-clinical-psychology/; retrieved 28 August 2015).

Perhaps related to the fuzziness of the distinction between CP and clinical psychology *as they are practiced* is the fact that although APA's Standards for Accreditation allow academic programs to be accredited as counseling psychology and clinical psychology training programs, this specialty distinction is not recognized for internships. Indeed, graduates from programs in both specialties compete for internships that are accredited in general *health service psychology* (and undesignated as *clinical* or *counseling* psychology). The umbrella term of health service psychologist includes individuals who have completed doctoral-level training in counseling, clinical, and school psychology programs that are accredited by the APA (1996).

Additionally, CP's relationship with *counseling* always has been close. CP shares with counseling many historical roots, perhaps more so than is the case with clinical psychology. In CP's early years, counseling psychologists often served in leadership roles in both the American Personnel and Guidance Association (APGA, now the American Counseling Association; ACA) and Division 17 (Goodyear, 2000). In contrast to Division 17 (the Society of Counseling Psychology) whose membership consists of approximately 2000 members, the ACA has more than 56,000 members, representing counseling in the US. Although there is much less cross-over in membership between the ACA and SCP than had previously been the case, some still exists. This is especially true for CP faculty who teach in master's degree programs in mental health counseling and want to model professional commitment to their students.

Licensure of CPs

In the US, the practice of psychology is regulated by individual states through a process of licensure. Although the APA (through CRSPPP) has worked to assist the public and the profession in differentiating among specialties in professional psychology, in most states, people are licensed simply as *psychologists*, regardless of their specialty or training background. Once licensed, they then are free to indicate their specialty or specialties if they choose. As Table 8 in Goodyear et al. (in press) shows, many CPs (36.4%) choose not to identify by specialty and represent themselves broadly as psychologists.

Although licensing requirements vary from state to state, the Association of State and Provincial Psychology Boards (ASPPB) works with states to ensure common standards, and some level of between-state licensure reciprocity. Among the common standards instantiated across states, is the requirement that to be licensed as a psychologist, the applicant must have completed a doctorate – generally a PhD, PsyD, or EdD – in psychology or a "closely related area." The doctoral degree must be from an APA-accredited program or one that is deemed an acceptable equivalent and the applicant must pass the Examination for the Professional Practice in Psychology (EPPP). Most states also require the completion of a full-time pre-doctoral internship and one year of postdoctoral clinical experience (Association of State and Provincial Psychology Boards [ASPPB], 2010).

In the 1970s, as licensure and the regulation of the practice of psychology became increasingly important in the US, the fact that many licensure statutes permitted individuals holding doctorates outside of psychology (but in "closely related areas") to become licensed as a psychologist became objectionable to the profession, and lobbying efforts were directed to states to eliminate that language which had been used as "a back door" through which individuals who were not trained in psychology (notably, those with degrees in counseling or counselor education) were able to obtain a psychology license. When licensure laws were rewritten and that metaphorical door was closed, many programs that had been offering a doctorate in counseling or counselor education became programs in counseling psychology.

Moreover, whereas, the number of APA-accredited CP programs had remained quite constant at about 23 for 25 years (from 1953, when the first programs were accredited, until 1978), the numbers began to grow steadily after those many counseling doctoral programs became programs in CP. Those numbers continued to rise for the next two decades, after which point they generally plateaued (Blustein, Goodyear, Perry, & Cypers, 2005). At present, there are 71 accredited CP programs and an additional seven that are *combined programs* (meaning that the programs focus on some combination of CP training along with training in either clinical or school psychology or both) (see http://apps.apa.org/accredsearch/). One challenge in the US has been that a number of research universities have closed their counseling psychology programs – even programs with very long and influential histories (e.g. Ohio State University; one of the two University of Minnesota programs) – though the number of accredited programs remains relatively constant, as new programs in universities that are less research focused are replacing the discontinued programs (Blustein et al., 2005).

Professional organizations

The specialty of CP is broadly represented in the US by the Counseling Psychology Specialty Council, which comprised representatives from 10 stakeholder organizations that collaboratively determine the dominant views and practices of CP (see http://cospp.org/specialties/counseling-psychology). The largest and most prominent stakeholder group is the Society of Counseling Psychology (SCP), which is a division (Division 17) of the APA. SCP has a membership of approximately 2000 members and affiliates and within it, there are 14 subspecialty sections (e.g. ethnic and racial diversity, supervision, and training) and 9 special interest groups (e.g. military issues, religious, and spiritual issues). The membership of SCP, however, reflects only a subset of the approximately

10,000 APA members who hold terminal degrees in CP (Lichtenberg, Goodyear, Overland, & Hutman, 2014).

CP is also represented by the American Academy of Counseling Psychologists (AACoP), whose membership comprised approximately 200 licensed psychologists who are board certified in CP by the American Board of Professional Psychology (ABPP). A third organization representing CP is the Council of Counseling Psychology Training Programs (CCPTP) – a group of approximately 75 doctoral training programs in counseling psychology, most of which are accredited by the APA. This organization, which focuses on training issues related to the professional preparation of CP graduates for positions in practice and academic settings, is independent of the Society of Counseling Psychology, but because of its role in the preparation of CPs, its decisions, actions and policy affect the entire specialty.

Where counseling psychologists work

As can be seen in Table 5 in Goodyear et al. (in press), the majority (59.0%) of those US CPs who are members of SCP are engaged in the provision of counseling or psychotherapy. Reported in more detail by Lichtenberg et al. (2014), CPs work in a variety of settings, including private practice, university counseling centers, VA medical centers, general and psychiatric hospitals, community mental health centers, and outpatient clinics. As described by the Society of Counseling Psychology in its statement to CRSPPP, the problems addressed by CP (and so, its role within the health care system) include, but are not limited to:

> educational and vocational/career/work adjustment concerns; vocational choice, and school-work-retirement transitions; relationship difficulties-including marital and family difficulties; learning and skill deficits; stress management and coping; organizational problems; adaptation to physical disabilities, disease, or injury; posttraumatic stress; personal/social adjustment; personality dysfunction; and mental disorders. (http://www.div17.org/wp-content/uploads/2012-CRSPPP-PETITION-w-Appendix.pdf; retrieved 28 August 2015)

It should be noted that even though many reported providing clinical services, the proportion of US CPs who serve *primarily* as practitioners was only 32.8%, whereas 41.3% of the US respondents indicated serving primarily as academicians (see Table 4 in Goodyear et al., in press). This finding may, in part, reflect the fact that membership in SCP (which was the population from which the sample of US CPs was drawn) is heavily represented by those working in academic settings. Indeed, Table 3 in Goodyear et al. (in press) shows that 55.7% of the US respondents indicated working as faculty primarily in universities or professional schools, more than double the highest proportion of that found in any of the other participating countries.

Traditions and core values

Despite the considerable overlap in the training and practices between clinical and counseling psychology (and between counseling psychology and counseling), CP traditions and core values are seen as uniquely defining features of the specialty. These traditions and values are listed in Table 10 of Goodyear et al. (in press). Data in that table indicate that US CPs most highly rated the values of attention to people's strengths and assets, and attention to diversity. Generally corroborating those results was Neimeyer and Diamond's (2001) finding the expert US CPs rated diversity highest among their list of values (attention to strengths was not an option).

US CP traces its roots back to career counseling, and especially to the work of Frank Parson (1909). Moreover, vocational psychology remains a strong strand within CP; it is counseling psychologists who have developed most major models of career counseling, and career counseling is an expected component of CP training (Murdock, Alcorn, Heesacker, & Stoltenberg, 1998; also see CCPTP's revised model training guidelines at http://www.ccptp.org/ccptp-model-training-program-guidelines). Given this historic centrality of career counseling in US CP, it was interesting (Table 10; Goodyear et al., in press) that US CPs rated this as 9th highest of 10 values. Apparently, this finding reflects a drift away from career counseling by most US CPs as the specialty evolves.

Another tradition or value of CP is its focus on the relationship as a primary vehicle of personal and therapeutic change. In this regard, the writings of Carl Rogers (1957) have been highly influential in the development and current status of US CP. This focus on the relationship in counseling and psychotherapy is especially prominent in CP's embrace of the "common factors" view of psychotherapy, or what Wampold and Imel (2015) refer to as the contextual model.

As noted earlier, CP training initially was to be grounded in a "scientist-practitioner" model and therefore the expected degree was the PhD Although this model continues to be the predominant one among US CP programs, an increasing number of programs now endorse a "practitioner-scholar" training model, preparing graduates specifically for practice careers and conferring a doctorate in psychology (PsyD). Coinciding with this evolution in training focus has been the already-noted attrition of CP programs in research universities and the growth of newer CP programs in regional universities and colleges (Blustein et al., 2005).

Challenges for CP in the US

Contemporary US CP faces a number of challenges. One is the declining number of individuals who are trained as CPs but who do not professionally affiliate with the specialty. The proportion of APA members who join most divisions is dropping, and this is reflected as well in the slow but steady drop in SCP membership, even though more than 300 new counseling psychologists graduate yearly. Relatedly, of the approximately 2000 members of SCP (which represents only about 20% of those members of APA whose degrees are in CP), only about 200 have elected to become board certified in the specialty – even though the majority of these APA/SCP member CPs are practitioners for whom specialty board certification would be expected to have career benefits. CRSPPP, as well as the American Board of Professional Psychology, have taken note of this fact and have questioned whether there is sufficient interest in CP to warrant its continued recognition as a professional specialty.

Another threat relates to restrictive rules that the Council for the Accreditation of Counseling and Related Educational Programs (CACREP) is imposing for the accreditation of counseling programs and the extent to which counseling licensure boards are insisting that licensure candidates graduate from CACREP accredited programs. Though supportive of recognizing program excellence among master's programs, CP has been challenged and threatened by accreditation standards for professional counseling programs that do not recognize CPs as legitimate core instructional faculty in those programs. The threat comes in two forms. First, whereas about 25% of US CP programs are housed in departments of psychology, most are in schools or colleges of education and have affiliated master's degree programs upon which they depend for tuition. CACREP's restrictive rules and the extent to which counseling licensure boards adopt CACREP as a standard, could endanger those master's programs, and therefore the CP programs associated with them. The second form of this threat concerns the employability of CP program graduates who otherwise would aspire to become faculty members in counseling programs or to become clinical supervisors for counselors. As we write this paper, these issues are especially prominent.

Conclusion

The specialty of SP in the US has undergone many developments and challenges since its inception in the early 1950s. This article has attempted to situate such developments and challenges in the US context by discussing how country-specific factors have influenced both the training and work of CPs over the years. It is our hope that counseling psychology will continue to thrive as a specialty with unique values and diverse functions.

Disclosure statement

No potential conflict of interest was reported by the authors.

References

Albee, G. W. (1998). Fifty years of clinical psychology: Selling our soul to the devil. *Applied and Preventive Psychology, 7,* 189–194.

American Psychological Association. (1996). *Recognition of health service providers.* Approved Council Resolution. C(17). Retrieved from http://www.apa.org/about/policy/chapter-10.aspx#recognition-service

American Psychological Association. Division Counseling and Guidance, Committee on Counselor Training. (1952a). Recommended standards for training counseling psychologists at the doctorate level. *American Psychologist, 7,* 175–181.

American Psychological Association. Division Counseling and Guidance, Committee on Counselor Training. (1952b). The practicum training of counseling psychologists. *American Psychologist, 7,* 182–188.

American Psychological Association. Division of Counseling Psychology, Committee on Definition. (1956). Counseling psychology as a specialty. *American Psychologist, 11,* 282–285.

American Psychological Association, Committee on Professional Standards (1981). Specialty Guidelines for the Delivery of Services by Counseling Psychologists. Washington, DC: APA.

Association of State and Provincial Psychology Boards. (2010). *ASPPB model act for licensure of psychologists*. Montgomery, AL: Author. Retrieved from https://asppb.site-ym.com/resource/resmgr/guidelines/final_approved_mlra_november.pdf

Blocher, D. H. (2000). *The evolution of counseling psychology*. New York, NY: Springer.

Blustein, D. L., Goodyear, R. K., Perry, J. C., & Cypers, S. (2005). The shifting sands of counseling psychology programs' institutional contexts: An environmental scan and revitalizing strategies. *The Counseling Psychologist, 33*, 610–634.

Dewsbury, D. A. (1999). Introduction. In D. A. Dewsbury (Ed.), *Unification through division: Histories of the divisions of the American Psychological Association* (Vol. III). (pp. 1–7). Washington, DC: American Psychological Association.

Gelso, C. J., Williams, E. N., & Fretz, B. R. (2014). *Counseling psychology* (3rd ed.). Washington, DC: American Psychological Association.

Goodyear, R. K. (2000). An unwarranted escalation of counselor-counseling psychologist professional conflict: Comments on Weinrach, Lustig, Chan, and Thomas (1998). *Journal of Counseling & Development, 78*, 103–106.

Goodyear, R. K., Lichtenberg, J. W., Hutman, H., Overland, E., Bedi, R., Christiani, K., … Young, C. (in press). A global portrait of counselling psychologists' characteristics, perspectives, and professional behaviors. *Counselling Psychology Quarterly*. doi: 10.1080/09515070.2015.1128396

Heppner, P. P., & Neal, G. W. (1983). Holding up the mirror: Research on the roles and functions of counseling centers in higher education. *The Counseling Psychologist, 11*, 81–98.

Lichtenberg, J. W., Goodyear, R. K., Overland, E. A., & Hutman, H. B. (2014, March). A snapshot of counseling psychology: Stability and change in the roles, identities and functions (2001–2014). *Presentation at the Counseling Psychology National Conference*, Atlanta, GA.

Munley, P. H., Duncan, L. E., Mcdonnell, K. A., & Sauer, E. M. (2004). Counseling psychology in the United States of America. *Counselling Psychology Quarterly, 17*, 247–271.

Murdock, N. L., Alcorn, J., Heesacker, M., & Stoltenberg, C. (1998). Model training program in counseling psychology. *The Counseling Psychologist, 26*, 658–672.

Neimeyer, G. J., & Diamond, A. K. (2001). The anticipated future of counselling psychology in the United States: A Delphi poll. *Counselling Psychology Quarterly, 14*, 49–65.

Parson, F. (1909). *Choosing a vocation*. Boston, MA: Houghton-Mifflin.

Raimy, V. C. (1950). *Training in clinical psychology*. Englewood Cliffs, NJ: Prentice Hall.

Rogers, C. R. (1957). The necessary and sufficient conditions of therapeutic personality change. *Journal of Consulting Psychology, 21*, 95–103.

Super, D. E. (1955). Transition: from vocational guidance to counseling psychology. *Journal of Counseling Psychology, 2*, 3–9.

Thompson, A. S., & Super, D. E. (1964). *The professional preparation of counseling psychologists* (Report of the 1964 Greyston Conference). New York, NY: Teachers College Press.

Wampold, B. E., & Imel, Z. E. (2015). The great psychotherapy debate (2nd ed.). New York: Routledge.

Weigel, R. G. (1977). I have seen the enemy and they is us and everyone else. *The Counseling Psychologist, 7*, 50–53.

Weissberg, M., Rude, S. S., Gazda, G. M., Bozarth, J. D., McDougal, K. S., Slavit, M. R., … Walsh, D. J. (1988). An overview of the third national conference for counseling psychology: Planning the future. *The Counseling Psychologist, 16*, 325–331.

Counselling psychology's genotypic and phenotypic features across national boundaries

Heidi Hutman[a], James W. Lichtenberg[b], Rodney K. Goodyear[c], Emily A. Overland[b]
and Terence J. G. Tracey[d]

[a]Division of Counseling Psychology, University at Albany, State University of New York, Albany, NY, USA; [b]Department of Educational Psychology, University of Kansas, Lawrence, KS, USA; [c]Graduate Department of Leadership and Counseling, University of Redlands, Redlands, CA, USA; [d]Counseling and Counseling Psychology, Arizona State University, Tempe, AZ, USA

This article integrates the survey results presented in the introductory article of this journal issue as well as the articles describing counselling psychology in each of the countries covered in the issue to examine the international character of counselling psychology. Specifically, it addresses the similarities and differences in the histories, education and training, demographics, and practice characteristics of the specialty within and across these national boundaries. The article concludes with an analysis of the value dimensions describing the international character of counselling psychology and addresses where the different countries place themselves along the two dimensions that were identified: Dimension 1 capturing basic research as different from most of the other values, and Dimension 2 being defined by an applied client focus versus a more indirect clinical perspective (i.e. social justice and research adding to the knowledge base).

The purpose of this special issue was to provide a cross-national snapshot of the characteristics of counselling psychologists, as well as to describe their professional roles, activities and values. The introductory article presented survey data from the eight participating countries: the United States (US), Canada, South Korea, South Africa, the United Kingdom (UK) of Great Britain, Australia, New Zealand and Taiwan. Each country then provided a narrative account of its respective survey results that highlighted the influence of country-specific factors on the nature and scope of counselling psychology. The goal of this article is to integrate the findings and observations reported in those preceding articles. More specifically, it attempts to pull together the information from the different countries in order to facilitate an understanding of what differentiates and unifies counselling psychologists globally. To this end, key differences and similarities will be discussed, followed by an interpretation of a correspondence analysis comparing the extent to which the eight countries varied in their endorsement of the specialty's core values.

Differences

Training and education

Differences across countries in the level of training and education required to be recognized as a counselling psychologist were found. Although all countries require graduate training in psychology, they differ with respect to whether a doctoral degree is required or whether a master's degree is sufficient. As Goodyear et al. (in press), reported, a doctoral degree from a specialty programme is required to practice in the US as a counselling psychologist, whereas in South Africa, New Zealand, Taiwan, South Korea, the UK and Australia, a master's degree in psychology (or alternative non-doctoral pathway) can be adequate. In Canada, the picture is more complex, as the educational level required to become a psychologist varies according to provincial regulations, with some provinces (e.g. British Columbia) requiring a doctoral degree and others (e.g. Alberta) deeming a master's degree to be sufficient professional training to perform the functions of a psychologist (Bedi, Sinacore, & Christiani, in press).

Age

The average age of counselling psychologists who responded to the surveys ranged from late thirties to mid-fifties across the eight countries, with South Korean respondents being the youngest ($M = 37.7$, $SD = 8.5$), and Australian respondents the oldest ($M = 55.1$, $SD = 12.0$). Interestingly, respondents' ages appeared to interact with their gender. For the most part, countries with older respondents (e.g. US) also tended to have larger percentages of males in their samples relative to countries with younger respondents (e.g.

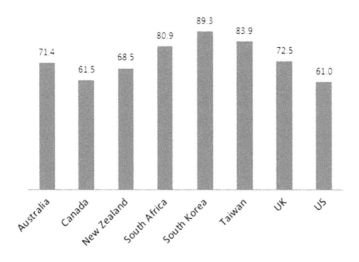

Figure 1. Proportion of female counselling psychologists by country.

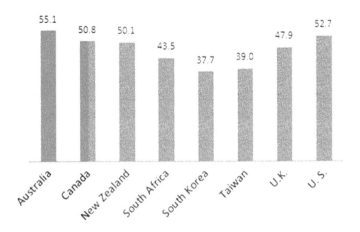

Figure 2. Mean age of counselling psychologists by country.

Taiwan). This trend is made especially clear when Figure 1 (proportion of women by country) and Figure 2 (mean age by country) are compared to one another.

It is also notable that counselling psychologists in Asia seem to be significantly younger than those practising in the other countries. To some extent, these differences in age and in the proportions of women seemed to reflect the length of the specialty's history in the particular countries.

Work settings, roles and activities

Diversity was observed in terms of the primary work settings and roles of counselling psychologists, as well as the extent to which they reported engaging in key activities. Whereas a sizeable group of counselling psychologists in Australia (47.4%), South Africa (47.3%), Canada (35.9%), the UK (32.3%) and New Zealand (29.6%) reported that they were either self-employed or in private practice, no respondents from South Korea or Taiwan indicated these settings as their primary working settings. In the latter counties, it seems to be more common for counselling psychologists to practice primarily in university counselling centres (South Korea: 23.2%, Taiwan: 28.2%). This finding may be attributed to the specialty in South Korea and Taiwan having early roots in educational settings (Ju, Han, Lee, & Lee, in press; Tu & Jin, in press). Furthermore, substantially more Taiwanese counselling psychologists (28.2%) indicated working in K-12 settings relative to the other participating countries, which makes sense in the context of the country's historical focus on assisting youth, as evidenced by the significance of the Teacher Chang Youth Guidance Center (Tu & Jin, in press).

Respondents in the US stood out, in that they were substantially more likely to indicate that they are university faculty than were their counterparts in the other countries. As Lichtenberg, Goodyear, Overland, and Hutman (2014) point out, the large proportion of counselling psychologists in academic settings reflects unique characteristics of society of counseling psychology (SCP) members, and is not necessarily representative of all professionals who identify as counselling psychologists. In fact, when the authors considered counselling psychologists who were non-SCP members, a clear majority of them indicated being self-employed or in private practice. In the UK, a significant percentage of respondents (31.2%) reported being primarily employed in the National Health Service, a reflection of employment challenges and pressures to reduce the cost of services there (Jones Nielsen & Nicholas, in press). Finally, the survey responses suggested considerable range in the occupational titles used to describe the primary work settings across countries, as captured by the "other" category. Thus, even though the functions are largely the same, country-specific differences in the language used to label positions were apparent.

Differences also were found among the eight countries in terms of counselling psychologists' primary work roles. The most pronounced differences seemed evident with the consultant, supervisor and academician roles: The proportions of counselling psychologists who endorsed consultant as their primary role ranged from 0.5 to 14% (UK). Across all countries, serving as a supervisor as one's primary work role was rare, with the highest proportion (Taiwan) being 3.3%. Furthermore, respondents from Canada and the US were most likely to indicate that they worked primarily as academicians (23.4 and 41.3%, respectively), whereas this proportion was 7.3% or less for half of the participating countries. Such differences could reflect characteristics of the job market that are unique to each country, or sample-specific idiosyncrasies, or most plausibly, both.

When respondents were asked about their engagement in key activities, the eight countries also exhibited wide variability. Although for most countries, a large proportion (44.9–69.8%) of counselling psychologists reported providing clinical supervision, the numbers were substantially lower in Taiwan and the UK (15.3 and 19.4%, respectively). Additionally, Taiwanese counselling psychologists who responded to the survey were unique, in that very few of them reported engaging in research-related activities relative to respondents from the other countries. The scarcity of Taiwanese counselling psychologists who conduct research seems reasonable in the context of respondents' low satisfaction ratings with their training in research and the lack of perceived value ascribed to engaging in research (Tu & Jin, in press) and the predominance of masters-level members of the specialty. Finally, South Korean counselling psychologists were much more likely to indicate that they were involved in assessment, which may be attributed to the fact that a specialized accredited training programme in psychologist assessment is offered (Ju et al., in press).

Contextual factors

This discussion of differences would be incomplete without addressing the impact of each country's particular national context on the development of the specialty, as well as contemporary issues that counselling psychologists face. The contributors all identified historical factors that have influenced the emergence of the specialty in their respective countries. For example, in the US, Second World War and the need for professionals who were trained to assist returning veterans provided the impetus for the introduction of specialty (Goodyear et al., in press). Alternatively, in New Zealand, du Preez, Feather, and Farrell (in press) trace the specialty's early origins to the native peoples, the Māori. The need for psychologists who could work with the White Afrikaans-speaking minority population was pivotal to the development of the specialty in South Africa (Bantjes, Kagee, & Young, in press). Thus, the history of the specialty is inextricably related to each country's respective context.

Similarly, the issues that counselling psychologists in each country face presently are linked to unique social, political and economic factors. As discussed above, pressures to provide low-cost services as well as limited employment options have led many counselling psychologists in the UK to work for the National Health Service (Jones Nielsen & Nicholas, in press). In South Korea, generational differences in the internalization of Confucian vs. Western values influence how counselling psychologists practice (Ju et al., in press). As a final example, the increasing popularity of the specialty and accompanying number of specialty programmes in Taiwan has led to concerns about whether the quality of training will be compromised and the job market will become oversaturated (Tu & Jin, in press).

Commonalities

Gender

All of the eight countries that contributed to this special issue have several characteristics that counselling psychologists share in common. One is the predominance of females. Cross-nationally, the overwhelming majority of survey respondents in each of the countries identified as female, with percentages ranging from 61% (US) to 89.3% (South Korea). As noted above, this trend is likely to persist, and even strengthen, as new generations of counselling psychologists enter the profession. Whether the changes in gender representation will influence the nature and scope of the specialty is an interesting question for future inquiry.

Work roles and activities

Although diversity was observed in terms of survey respondents' primary work roles and engagement in key activities, similarities also were apparent across countries. When asked about their primary work roles, over half of the respondents in all but one of the countries indicated that they worked primarily as clinical practitioners. Taiwanese counselling psychologists were the exception, albeit a fairly significant proportion (21%) of respondents still endorsed this category. It was also rare for counselling psychologists from all participating countries to indicate serving primarily as administrators, researchers and academicians.

Nevertheless, across the eight countries, most respondents indicated being involved in administrative tasks. This trend makes sense in light of these increasing emphases on accountability and accompanying paperwork demands for psychologists globally. Consistent with the pattern for the category of primary work roles, in all of the countries except Taiwan, most counselling psychologists reported providing counselling and psychotherapy, with percentages ranging from 59% (US) to an impressive 93.9% (South Korea). Again, a significant proportion of the Taiwanese respondents still indicated providing counselling and psychotherapy (36.1%), but the number was smaller relative to the other countries. In comparison to the other categories, fewer counselling psychologists appear to be engaged in career counselling and vocational assessment, based on the survey responses. Overall, the emphasis on clinical practice appears to transcend national boundaries and represents one way in which counselling psychologists around the world are similar.

Identity struggles

The struggle for counselling psychologists to differentiate themselves from clinical psychologists and other allied mental health subspecialties seems to be an international phenomenon, though manifesting itself in different forms depending on the national context. For example, in the US, clinical and counselling psychologists hold the same license and seem increasingly difficult to differentiate and until recently, accreditation procedures were the same for clinical psychology and counselling psychology programmes in Canada, which was viewed as a threat to the distinct professional identity of Canadian counselling psychologists (Bedi et al., in press; Sinacore, 2015; Young & Lalande, 2011).

In several countries, clinical psychologists hold a more privileged status. For example, in South Korea, clinical psychologists have statutory regulation, whereas counselling psychologists are regulated by professional associations (Ju et al., in press). Moreover, in some countries, clinical psychologists' more privileged status threatens the specialty's future. For example, in South Africa, only clinical psychologists can be employed in the state mental health system, which is contributing to a decline in the number of counselling programmes (Bantjes et al., in press). In Australia, the differential pay and responsibilities between clinical and counselling psychology is threatening the survival of the specialty (Di Mattia & Grant, in press). Whereas the New Zealand situation is similar to that of South Africa, in that only clinical psychologists can be employed in the health delivery system, the single specialty training programme is relatively new and circumstances might change as dialogues with clinical psychology continue.

Satisfaction

On a more positive note, when asked about their satisfaction with the specialty as a career choice and with their graduate training, respondents from all eight countries reported being highly satisfied. On a 6-point scale, ratings ranged by country from 4.09 to 5.51, with respondents giving slightly lower, but still high, ratings for satisfaction with their training relative to their career choice. Thus, in spite of their shared struggles for a distinct professional identity, counselling psychologists appear to feel quite positively about their career decisions and training.

Professional values

Respondents were asked to indicate their level of endorsement of professional values that are considered integral to the identity of counselling psychologists. Although each country modified the wording to be more consistent with how the profession is understood in their respective contexts, overall, the values emphasized: (a) a strengths-based perspective, (b) a developmental focus, (c) career counselling, (d) prevention, (e) using research to inform practice, (f) conducting research to add to the counselling psychology knowledge base, (g) short- and long-term interventions, (h) person-environment interactions, (i) diversity and multiculturalism and (j) social justice and advocacy. To assess the extent to which the eight countries differed and were similar in their endorsement of these values, a correspondence analysis was conducted.

Correspondence analysis (Greenacre, 2007; Weller & Romney, 1990), also called dual scaling (Nishisato, 1980) and canonical analysis of cross-classified data (Holland, Levi, & Watson, 1980), is analogous to conducting a principal-components analysis on a two-way frequency table. Dimensions are extracted separately for row and column variation. These dimensions can then be plotted together on a graph to represent their covariation with proximity representing similarity. These data were analysed using the R application CA, a software package that allows for the results of this analysis to be represented in two- and three-dimensional graphics (Nenadic & Greenacre, 2007). As in principal-components analysis, correspondence analysis computes eigenvalues (and percentage of variance accounted for [VAF]), which can then be used to determine the appropriate number of dimensions to interpret. Eigenvalues (VAFs follow in parentheses) of 0.0027 (64%), .0010 (21%) and .0003 (8%), were obtained for the first three components, and it is clear that the best structure was based on two components. The bi-plot of the values and the countries are presented in Figure 3.

The distances depicted in Figure 3 represent the relative similarity, with things graphed closer being more similar and things more distant being more dissimilar. This plot can be examined with regard to how similar values are to each other, how similar countries are to each other, and also how countries map onto the different values. For the values, Dimension 1 captures basic research as different from most all other values (with the possible exception of career), whereas Dimension 2 is defined by an applied client

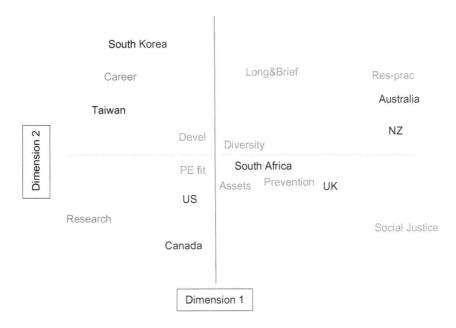

Figure 3. Bi-plot of the spatial representation of core values (in red) by country (in black). Abbreviations for core values: Assets = a strengths-based perspective, Devel = developmental focus, Career = career counselling, Prevention = prevention focus, Res-prac = using research to inform practice, Research = conducting research to add to the counselling psychology knowledge base, Long&Brief = short- and long-term interventions, PE fit = person-environment interactions, Diversity = diversity and multiculturalism, and Social justice = social justice and advocacy. Abbreviations for country: NZ = New Zealand, UK = United Kingdom, US = United States.

focus (short- and long-term interventions, developmental focus, career interventions, and using research to inform practice, and research aimed at aiding practice) versus a more indirect or less clinical perspective (i.e. social justice and research adding to the knowledge base). So the values focused on basic research versus practice, and individual client work versus more indirect work. Those values depicted in the middle (i.e. prevention, PE fit, Diversity and a strengths-based perspective) are viewed as similar to each other.

An examination of the plot of countries only demonstrates that factor 1 separates Taiwan and South Korea (and somewhat Canada and US) from New Zealand and Australia, and US Dimension 2 differentiates Canada (and to a lesser extent the UK) from Australia, Taiwan and South Korea. With reference just to proximity, Taiwan and South Korea are similar with respect to values as are Australia and New Zealand.

Examining values juxtaposed with countries gives an understanding regarding how the countries differ in values. Canada and, to a lesser extent, the US are separate with respect to their having the highest valuing of both basic research and social justice. Taiwan and South Korea have highest endorsement for basic research and a career focus. Taiwan and South Korea were the only countries that were close to career values at all. All other countries were plotted some distance away indicating that a career focus is not at all present among their core values. Australia and New Zealand were similar in their endorsement of research as a means of assisting practice and clear clinical applications with respect to short- and long-term interventions. The UK was more balanced with respect to their relative valuing of applied clinical focus versus social justice. Finally the Republic of South Africa was perhaps the most centrally placed country, and thus represents a relative balance among the values depicted.

Conclusion

Although each country's particular national context clearly has an influence on who counselling psychologists are and the professional functions they fulfill, there are also similar features that transcend international borders and provide a unified picture of the specialty. Based on the survey results from the eight contributing countries, the genotypic features of counselling psychologists are that they are most likely to be females who identify as practitioners and engage in clinical work and administrative tasks. Furthermore, regardless of their country of origin, they are united in their struggle to differentiate themselves from other mental health professionals and have a distinct identity. In other words, the unique national climate may shape the specialty's phenotypic presentation, but underneath, there is a shared gene pool that creates an international bond. We hope that this special issue facilitates an international understanding of the specialty and stimulates future collaborations among counselling psychologists around the world.

Disclosure statement

No potential conflict of interest was reported by the authors.

References

Bantjes, J., Kagee, A., & Young, C. (in press). Counselling psychology in South Africa. *Counselling Psychology Quarterly.* doi: 10.1080/09515070.2015.1128401

Bedi, R. P., Sinacore, A. L., & Christiani, K. D. (in press). Counselling Psychology in Canada. *Counselling Psychology Quarterly.* doi: 10.1080/09515070.2015.1128398

Di Mattia, M. A., & Grant, J. (in press). Counselling psychology in Australia: History, status, and challenges. *Counselling Psychology Quarterly.* doi: 10.1080/09515070.2015.1127208

du Preez, E., Feather, J., & Farrell, B. (in press). Counselling psychology in New Zealand. *Counselling Psychology Quarterly.* doi: 10.1080/09515070.2015.1128397

Goodyear, R. K., Lichtenberg, J. W., Hutman, H., Overland, E., Bedi, R., Christiani, K., ... Young, C. (in press). A global portrait of counselling psychologists' characteristics, perspectives, and professional behaviors. *Counselling Psychology Quarterly.* 10.1080/09515070.2015.1128396

Greenacre, M. J. (2007). *Correspondence analysis in practice* (2nd ed.). Boca Raton, FL: Chapman & Hall/CRC.

Holland, T. R., Levi, M., & Watson, C. G. (1980). Canonical correlation in the analysis of a contingency table. *Psychological Bulletin, 87*, 334–336. doi:10.1037/0033-2909.87.2.334

Jones Nielsen, J. D., & Nicholas, H. (in press). Counseling psychology in the United Kingdom. *Counselling Psychology Quarterly.* doi: 10.1080/09515070.2015.1127210

Ju, Y. A., Han, Y., Lee, H., & Lee, D. Y. (in press). Counselling psychology in South Korea. *Counselling Psychology Quarterly.* doi: 10.1080/09515070.2015.1127209

Lichtenberg, J. W., Goodyear, R. K., Overland, E. A., & Hutman, H. (2014, March). *A snapshot of counseling psychology: Stability and change in the roles, identities and functions (2001–2014).* Presented at the National Conference on Counseling Psychology, Atlanta, GA.

Nenadic, O., & Greenacre, M. (2007). Correspondence analysis in R, with two- and three-dimensional graphics: The CA package. *Journal of Statistical Software, 20*(3), 1–13.

Nishisato, S. (1980). *Analysis of categorical data: Dual scaling and its applications.* Toronto: University of Toronto Press.

Sinacore, A. L. (2015). Introduction. In A. L. Sinacore & F. Ginsberg (Eds.), *Canadian counselling and counselling psychology in the 21st century* (pp. 3–14). Montreal: McGill-Queens University Press.

Tu, S. F., & Jin, S. R. (in press). Development and current status of counselling psychology in Taiwan. *Counselling Psychology Quarterly.* doi: 10.1080/09515070.2015.1128399

Weller, S. C., & Romney, A. K. (1990). *Metric scaling: Correspondence analysis.* Sag University Paper Series on Quantitative Applications in the Social Sciences, Series No. 07-075. Newbury Park, CA: Sage.

Young, R. A., & Lalande, V. (2011). Canadian counselling psychology: From defining moments to ways forward. *Canadian Psychology/Psychologie Canadienne, 52*, 248–255. doi:10.1037/a0025165

Index

INDEX

private health insurance 30
private practice 8, 26–7, 87, 92, 111–12
professional identity 13, *14–15*, 40–1
professional organizations 93, 104–5
professional school faculties 8
psychiatric hospitals 41
psychodynamic model 27
psychological displacement paradigm of diary
  writing (PDPD) 88
Psychological Society of SA (PsySSA),
  Association for CP 58
psychological therapy 25, 28–30; community
  interventions 60–1; hybrid interventions 60
Psychologist, The 91
Psychologists Act (Taiwan, 2001) 79–88; CP
  and CT separation and identity formation
  81–3, *82–3*; Enforcement Rules 84–5;
  examinations and internship programmes
  83–5; legislation stage 80–3; post-legislation
  stage 84; pre-legislation stage 79–80; and
  quality assurance 85
Psychology Board of Australia (PsyBA) 24–5;
  area of endorsement 24, 29; *Guidelines on*
  area of practice endorsements 29
psychopathology, and well-being distinction 58
psychotherapy 27, 50, 73

Qualification in Counselling Psychology
  (QCoP) 93–4; *Enrolment Guidelines* 94
Qualification Standards Committee (UK) 94
quality assurance 85
Quality Assurance Agency (UK) 94; Subject
  Benchmark Statement for Psychology 94
Queensland University (Brisbane) 24

racial exclusion 63
Reality Dynamic Counseling 74
reflective practitioner model 95
refugees 63
registration 24–5, 30, 36, 58, 61, 70, 75; options
  (Australia) 24; race and gender (South
  Africa) 61, *62*; requirements (New Zealand)
  48–9
Regulations Regarding Study and Counselling
  Assistance for Overseas Chinese Students
  (Taiwan) 79
rehabilitation centers 41
relationship counselling centers 26–7, 74
remedial interventions 73
research 38
resources 61
Rhee, D. 69
Rose Committee report (Australia, 1970) 23

Scherman, R., and Feather, J. 50
Schoenberg, M. 35

schools 41, 57, 73
scientist–practitioner model 95, 106
scope of practice (SoP) 47, 58, 61, 82
Section of Counselling Psychology (SCP,
  Canada) 34–8, 42–4; Archive Committee 36;
  Definition Committee 36
self-employed 8, 92, 111–12
self-identity 40
self-regulating organizations 30
Seo, Y.S., *et al.* 76
Seoul Board of Education 68–9
Seul, C.-D., Bae, J.-W. and Cheon, S.-M. 69
Sinacore, A. 36; Christiani, K. and Bedi, R.
  34–46
Smith, D., and Lancaster, S. 26
social justice 38, 59–60
social services 57, 87
social workers 73
Society for Counseling Psychology (SCP, NZ)
  20
Society of Counseling Psychology (SCP, US)
  111; APA Division 17 5, 103–6
South African Journal of Psychology (SAJP)
  58
South African Psychology Congress 58
Square for Youth's Conversation 69
Standards of Proficiency (SOP) 91
Stellenbosch University 55
stigma 59, 62
substance abuse 59
suicide rates 75
Super, D. 1, 15
surveys 2–20; career choice satisfaction 15, *16*,
  114; contextual factors 112–13; core values
  15–19, *17–19*, 38–40, 50–1, 72–4, 105–6,
  114–16, **115**; countries included 2–5, 109–16;
  demographic information 5–8, *6–7*, 110–13,
  110–11; discussion 19–20; method 3–5;
  perspectives, beliefs and attitudes 13, 74;
  professional identity 13–15, *14–15*, 40–1, 74,
  81–3, *82–3*; 74-item questionnaire 34–5;
  work settings, roles and activities 8–12,
  9–12, 86–7, 92–3, *93*, 105, 111–13
Swinburne University of Technology
  (Melbourne) 24
systemic model 27
Systems theories 41

T-groups 69
Taipei Counselling Psychologists Association
  4, 86
Taiwan 79–88; Bureau of Education 79;
  Counselling and Guidance Association
  (TGCA) 84–8; Counselling Psychologist
  Union (TCPU) 86; Counselling Psychology
  Association (TWCPA) and group members

123

For Product Safety Concerns and Information please contact our EU
representative GPSR@taylorandfrancis.com
Taylor & Francis Verlag GmbH, Kaufingerstraße 24, 80331 München, Germany

www.ingramcontent.com/pod-product-compliance
Ingram Content Group UK Ltd.
Pitfield, Milton Keynes, MK11 3LW, UK
UKHW031043080625
459435UK00013B/541